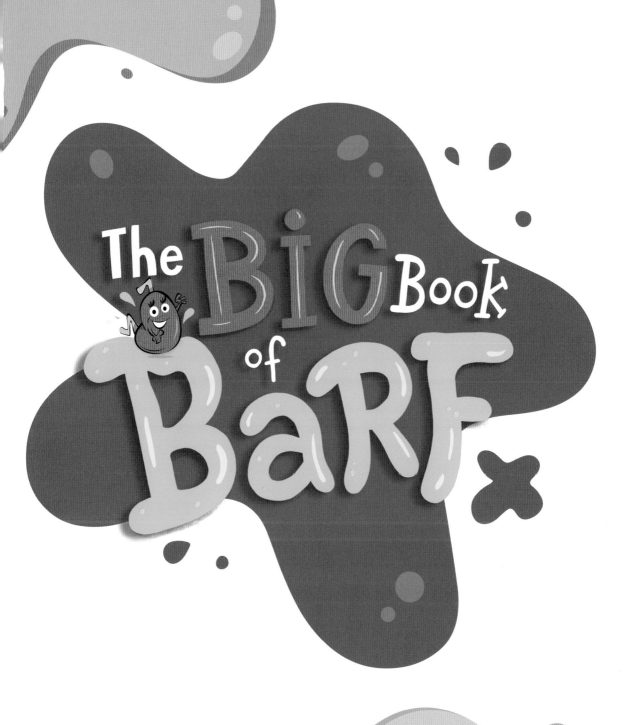

The BiG Book of BaRF

The BiG Book of BaRF

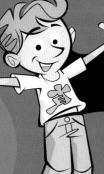

A SPEWNAMI of SICK SCIENCE, HURLED HISTORY, and BODY ODDITIES

Vicky Lorencen

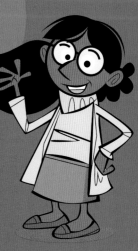

BRIGHT MATTER BOOKS

All rights reserved. Published in the United States by Bright Matter Books, an imprint of
Random House Children's Books, a division of Penguin Random House LLC, New York.

Bright Matter Books and colophon are registered trademarks
of Penguin Random House LLC.

Visit us on the Web! rhcbooks.com

Educators and librarians, for a variety of teaching tools,
visit us at RHTeachersLibrarians.com

Library of Congress Cataloging-in-Publication Data is available upon request.
ISBN 978-0-593-70791-3 (trade)—ISBN 978-0-593-70793-7 (lib. bdg.)—
ISBN 978-0-593-70792-0 (ebook)

The text of this book is set in 11-point Museo Slab 500 and 10-point Benton Sans Pro.
Interior design by Michelle Crowe
Cover design by April Ward

MANUFACTURED IN CHINA
10 9 8 7 6 5 4 3 2 1
First Edition

FOR MY HUSBAND,
WITH LOVE AND GRATITUDE.

YOU SAID THE WORD.

I SAID, "HEY! THAT COULD BE SOMETHING!"

AND LOOK WHERE WE ARE NOW.

(I SHOULD LISTEN TO YOU MORE OFTEN.)

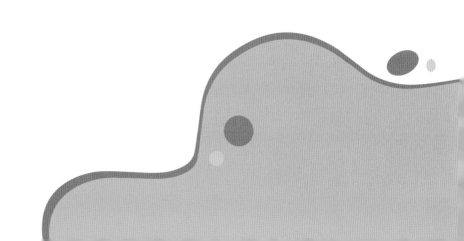

INTRODUCTION

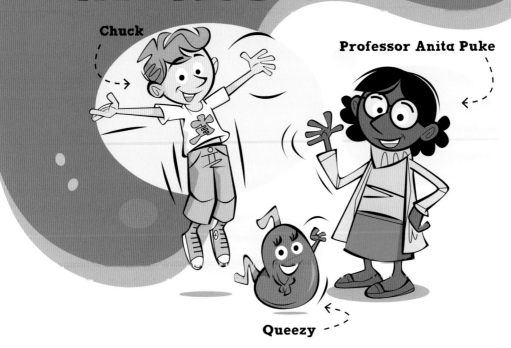

Chuck

Professor Anita Puke

Queezy

HI! I'M CHUCK. YUP. AS IN, UPCHUCK.

This is my sidekick in spew, Queezy.

Whether you call it vomit, barf, or the chunder from down under, this book is for kids like you and me who love gross the most. Hungry to know more about *hork*? A *spew*nami of sick science, Hurled History, Ralph-worthy Recipes (like Barfday Cake!), and glistening goo-formation overflow every puke-filled page. (Sorry if they're sticky.)

Curious to learn what *really* goes on in your innards? My pal Professor Anita Puke can stomach any question you heave her way. So don't hold it in! Trust me, Professor Puke knows vomit inside and out, from arf to zork. She's prepared to spill the soup about our amazing bodies and what they do to protect us—before we even know it!

Along our ralphabetical ramble through this book, Queezy will pick Professor Puke's mighty mind too. Queezy is always good for a belly laugh, and she has the guts to ask *anything*!

And hey, sure, it's called *The Big Book of Barf,* but you don't have to swallow this spewing spree of science and silly stuff in one big gulp. Pace yourself. Skip around. Explore. Check out one easy-to-digest chunk at a time. Let this barf-fet of gargle gravy goopness soak in.

When you reach the end of the ralphabet and peel back that last pukey page, surprise! The frothy face fountain of facts and fun is far from done. There's a "hurl" lot more!

You get a bonus sick sack of Back Splatter! It's a belly blow-out featuring a gloppy glossary, a map of all my insides, and 205 squirmy terms to make your vomit vocabulary explode. Plus, since bathrooms/barfrooms are the preferred place to puke, we've got words from around the world for that VIP (Very Important Place).

You ready to dive in?

We sure are!

Heave-ho! Let's go!

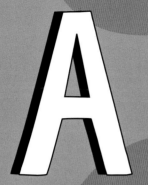

A

When it comes to your body and barf, your mind probably jumps to your middle section—better known as your **abdomen.** It's true. That area holds *a lot.* While we're down there, we'll get acquainted with awesome organs and how they function, dig into the differences between good and bad bacteria, and even pick the "pocket" of your digestive system (also known as your **appendix**).

Plus, we'll get the scoop on food **allergies,** and you'll learn how to make **Awesome Arf Meal.** This sick and simple spin on oatmeal from Queezy's uncle Urp makes the best barf-fest . . . if you can stomach it.

And away we go!

TURN UP THE VOLUME ON YOUR VOMIT VOCABULARY

After-Dinner Drainer: when dinner goes out of you after you go out to dinner

All-Out Spout: gush grape soda like a gloppy purple geyser

Animated Throat Missiles: launch a tummy tantrum into the toilet target

Arf: barf on all fours like a dog

Atomic Vomit: when goop explodes as the belly unloads

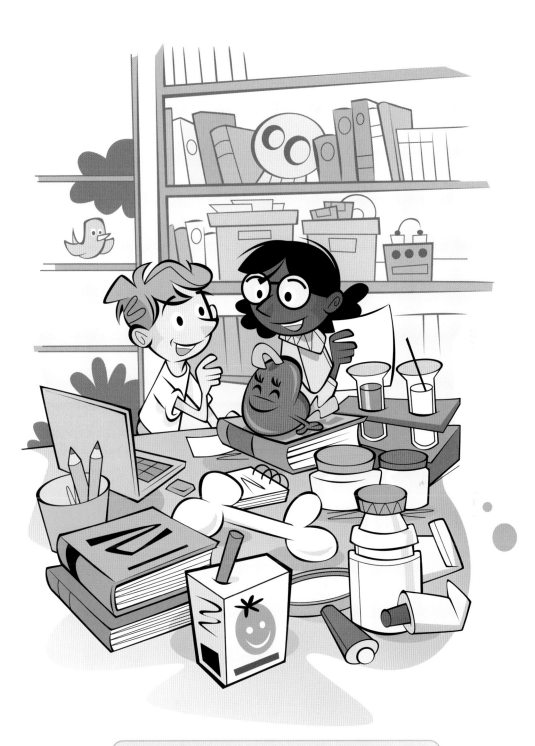

 CHUCK AND QUEEZY: Hi, Professor Puke! Queezy and I don't know anybody who knows more about atomic vomit than you.

QUEEZY: You're like the princess of puke to me!

 PROFESSOR ANITA PUKE: Hey, thanks! I do have a deep appreciation for the body's ability to protect itself, and sometimes that includes vomiting.

 CHUCK: I wonder if you know as many ways to say "vomit" as I do.

 I'm sure we can teach each other a *spew* things.

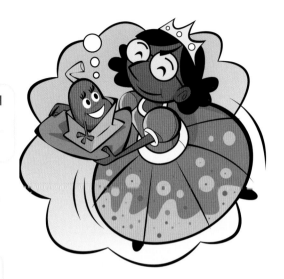

 Spew is right! That's why we're here. Queezy and I had the flu all last week.

 I'm sorry to hear that. Food flew right through you, didn't it?

 Yes! It was a real barf-athon. Why do our bodies reject stuff anyway?

I'd love to tell you. How about we begin from the inside out?

 Great! We have lots to ask you.

 Hurl those questions at me any time!

 Thank you, Princess—I mean, Professor! Hmm, where should we start?

How about ralphabetically, with letter A?

CHUCK'S SICK SCIENCE

A Is for Abdomen

 PROFESSOR ANITA PUKE: Your abdomen is the space between your ribs and your hips. Sandwiched in your abdomen are the digestive organs.

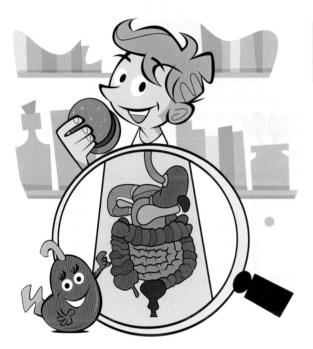

CHUCK: You're talking about the body parts that process stuff you slurp or poke down the shoot, like the cheeseburger I had for lunch.

QUEEZY: All I heard was sandwich and cheeseburger. Yum!

Let's take a quick tour of these, um, processors of stuff you poke down the shoot, as you put it. First, we see the stomach.

Oh! My favorite! The Puke Purse! The Barfpack! The Sick Sack!

 The stomach is one of the most important organs of the abdomen, especially where vomiting is concerned.

What's that thing tucked behind the stomach?

 That's the pancreas, and it makes a special enzyme. An enzyme is like a powerful juice that breaks down the fat and protein in the foods you eat.

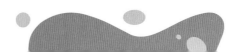

It's a Cheeseburger Disintegrator.

Isn't that amazing? Now let's meet the liver. It cleans the blood leaving the stomach and intestine. The liver also ships nutrients out to the rest of the body and saves some energy for later. Any leftover nutrients become a greenish-yellow digestive fluid called bile. Sometimes bile shows up in vomit.

 Cool. I'm calling that a Bile Burp!

After the liver makes bile, the bile is stored in the gallbladder. You can think of it like a bile warehouse. Then bile goes to the small intestine to help the body break down and soak up fat from the food for energy.

 Ooh. What are those two things? Big beans?

These beauties are the kidneys. This impressive pair removes waste products from your body. As a side job, they make it possible for your body to use vitamin D to grow strong bones.

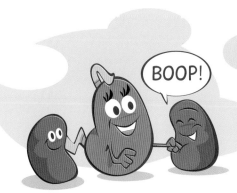

BOOP!

 Hey, thanks, Kidney Twins.

Next, we see the small intestine and the large intestine.

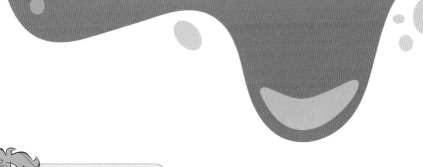

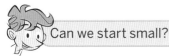
Can we start small?

Sure! The small intestine soaks up nutrients from your food, as well as water that will move into your bloodstream or be used for jobs like digesting food.

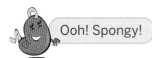
Ooh! Spongy!

Once the small intestine finishes its job, anything the body doesn't need heads to the large intestine, where it soaks up any water or leftover nutrients the small intestine sends its way. And that completes the inventory of the abdomen. So, there you go!

And speaking of "there you go," isn't the tail end of the large intestine where the "you know what" hangs out until you set it free?

The "you know what"?

Go ahead, say it.

Are you referring to feces?

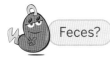
Feces?

Okay, then, excrement.

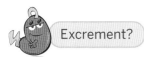
Excrement?

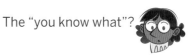

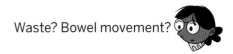

Waste? Bowel movement?

Come on, Professor Puke, please?

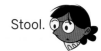

Stool.

POOP! You were supposed to say "poop"!

Very well The muscles in the rectum push the, uh, poop out of the body.

There you go! Well, not literally.

Hope you enjoyed that. You will never hear me say poop again.

Um, Professor Puke, you just did.

Ha! Why don't we push on to your next question?

Queezy's Question

Why do food allergies make you "all-out spout"?

PROFESSOR ANITA PUKE: Allergies can happen with all kinds of foods. For kids, foods like milk, eggs, and peanuts are the most common causes of a food allergy. If you eat a food you're allergic to, it can make your immune system go berserk.

QUEEZY: *Danger! Danger! Get that food out of here!*

Your immune system helps your body protect itself from outside invaders by sending antibodies to detect and tackle bad guys like germs that can make you sick. The immune system takes its job very seriously.

CHUCK: Sometimes too seriously?

When your immune system overreacts to a food, you might get an itchy, tingling feeling in your mouth, or you could break out in a rash, experience a swollen tongue or lips, or even have trouble breathing.

Wow. So that's what an allergic reaction feels like.

Maybe I shouldn't slurp an egg and peanut milkshake to test it out?

Trust your gut on that one, Queezy!

Can allergic reactions make you "all-out spout"?

They sure can.

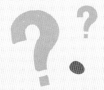 Hey, that's smart! If the body says no, then out it goes. Gross.

But smart.

CHUCK'S SICK SCIENCE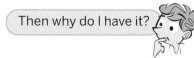

Dig Deep into the Pocket of Your Digestive System . . . Your Appendix

 PROFESSOR ANITA PUKE: Your appendix is a small pouch attached to the top of your large intestine.

 CHUCK: What's in the pouch? Candy bars? Quarters?

 For your sake, let's hope it's nothing.

What good is a pocket if you can't stuff your stuff in it?

 If your appendix gets blocked by "stuff"—like . . . poop— bad bacteria can grow and cause an infection called appendicitis.

You said poop again! But I'll pass on the poop pocket, thanks.

 Appendicitis pain usually begins around your belly button and moves down the right side of your abdomen. You'd probably have a fever, become nauseous, and vomit. An infected appendix could burst. People with appendicitis usually need an operation to remove their appendix.

Can I live without my appendix?

 Absolutely.

Then why do I have it?

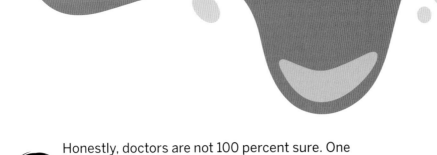

 Honestly, doctors are not 100 percent sure. One theory is that the appendix may store good gut bacteria.

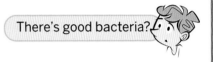 There's good bacteria?

 Yes! After you've been sick with something like norovirus, the digestive tract may use some of the healthy bacteria your appendix has tucked away to help get your gut back in shape.

So it's a battle of good guts versus bad guts?

 I would call it "bac"-to-"bac" combat! Your gut health is in the balance!

LEARN MORE about the trillions of micro-fighters in the gut by going to page 133.
No idea what norovirus is? Check out page 142.

Uncle Urp's Awesome Arf Meal

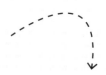

MAKES 2 SERVINGS

> **QUEEZY**: Yum. How's your appetite? Got room for something tasty? Then this Awesome Arf Meal is perfect for you! This simple spin on oatmeal comes topped with a delicate "bile" drizzle. You can have it any time of day, but I like it in the morning. It's the best *barf-fast* ever. Just like Uncle Urp used to make!

YOU WILL NEED:

- 1 cup dry traditional oatmeal*

- 2 cups milk (or water)

- Salt—just a dash (less than ⅛ teaspoon)

- ½ cup applesauce (chunky applesauce was Uncle Urp's favorite, but any kind will do)

- 1 drop green food coloring

*If you prefer to use instant oatmeal, skip steps 1 through 4 and instead follow the directions on the package. Once you've made your oatmeal, head to steps 5 and 6 to complete your meal.

⭐ **Before you begin:** Practice food safety (and avoid the vomit). Always start by washing your hands and cleaning the area of the kitchen where you'll be cooking. You'll want an adult to help you. Make sure your assistant has clean hands too!

HERE'S WHAT YOU NEED TO DO:

Step 1: Pour the milk or water into a pan and add a dash of salt. Ask your adult assistant to help place the pan on the stove and turn the burner on. Cook over medium-high heat until the liquid comes to a boil (meaning there are lots of bubbles—but don't let it bubble over).

Step 2: Stir in the oats.

Step 3: Turn down the heat to medium and continue cooking the oats for five minutes. Give the pan a stir every minute or two.

Step 4: After five minutes, take the pan off the heat and scoop the oatmeal into two bowls.

Step 5: In a separate bowl, mix the applesauce and green food coloring.

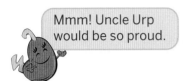

Mmm! Uncle Urp would be so proud.

Step 6: Use a spoon to drizzle the applesauce mixture over the oatmeal. Enjoy!

NOW THAT your belly is full of Uncle Urp's Awesome Arf Meal, you'd better pack bigger barf bags because letter B is brimming with brain benders. What's the big deal with balance, and why does it even matter? That answer may make your head bobble.

Believe it or not, just beyond this page, you'll behold a bizarre museum, baffling facts about burping, and a barfing black hole. Bonus! Get the backstory on a brilliant invention!

Let's bounce! Letter B is the place to "B."

B

Be prepared to behold the connection between **balance,** the ears, and one of the most common reasons to **"blow chunks."** But that's not all!

You'd better be ready for the bizarre! Ever heard of a magical **bezoar**? No? Okay, how about a **black hole** that barfs? Prepare to meet the hurling creator **Bumba,** and the dude who invented the handy-dandy **barf bag.**

Bonus! You'll be blown away (candles and all) by a Ralph-worthy Recipe for **Barfday Cake**!

TURN UP THE VOLUME ON YOUR VOMIT VOCABULARY

Barf: arf like a dog with bad breath

Bark at the Ants: end a picnic by barfing in the basket

Belly Blowout: when the belly fills up, the belly blows out

Belly Deli: purge a pastrami and salami tsunami

Belly Jelly: un-jam food sandwiched in the stomach

Blast the Bathroom: have a belly outburst

Blow Chunks: hurl a cottage cheese smoothie

Bomb the Bathroom: explode in the commode or go kaboom in the bathroom

Boomerang Breakfast: see the return of the scrambled eggs

Burst Your Belly Bubble: eat and eat until the belly pops and lunch leaks out

CHUCK'S SICK SCIENCE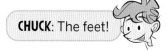

B Is for Balance

 PROFESSOR ANITA PUKE: Balance and motion sickness both begin in—

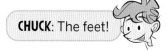 **CHUCK**: The feet!

 Sorry. Not even close. Balance and motion sickness both begin in the ears.

 What?! Did I hear you right? Are you trying to burst my belly bubble? Why are you talking about ears?

Trust me, there's a connection between ears and vomit. Let me explain. Your ears have three parts. Each part has its own job, but they work as a team. The outer ear (the part you can see on the outside of the head) pulls in sound and funnels it to the ear canal. The sound then slides into the middle ear.

 I'm glad it doesn't tickle.

 The middle ear turns those sound waves into vibrations and sends them over to the inner ear. The inner ear takes those vibrations and changes them into signals that go to the brain.

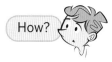 How?

 The inner ear has slim tubes filled with fluid and tiny hairs.

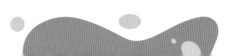

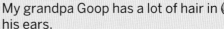 My grandpa Goop has a lot of hair in his ears.

 You can't see or feel the tiny hairs in the inner ear.

 How do I know the hairs are working?

 Let's try this. Stand back. Give yourself plenty of room. Stretch your arms out to the sides like airplane wings. Now spin around. Keep spinning until you've counted to ten Belly Blowouts.

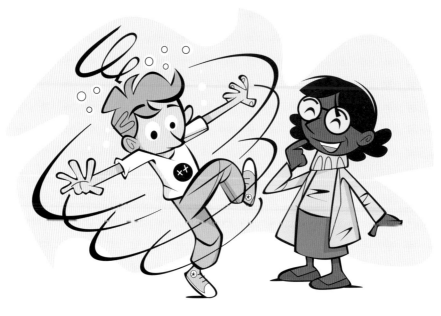

 Stop! I predict you're feeling dizzy and finding it hard to keep your balance.

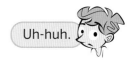 Uh-huh.

 You feel wobbly because the fluid in the inner ear is still sloshing around. The tiny hairs are telling your brain your body is still spinning. That confused, out-of-balance, "I'm moving but I'm standing still" feeling makes some people—

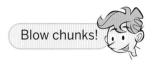
Blow chunks!

Better believe it! Motion sickness happens to about one in three people.

Aren't I lucky to be one of them . . .

The good news—your ears work!

THE BIZARRE BEZOAR

A *bezoar* is (usually) a blob of undigested food that hardens into a solid mass in the stomach or somewhere else in the digestive system.

Bezoars may cause nausea or even make you vomit. Or they can create real problems by keeping food trapped in your stomach when it should be moving into the small intestine and giving your body the nutrients it needs.

Bezoars are most often a conglomeration of food particles the body can't digest, like an apple stem, seeds, or pits. Other kinds of bezoars may be a gob of hair (from chewing on hair) and bits of food, or undigested milk and mucus. People who need to take medications like antacids due to a medical condition may have a bezoar "meatball" made of undigested pills and the capsules the medication comes in.

Before you get yourself wrapped in a ball of worry, bezoars are not common. For example, a busy hospital might see fewer than three patients with a bezoar in a whole year.

Bezoar Magic

It's believed the word *bezoar* comes from an Arabic word—*badzehr*—or from a Persian word—*padzhar*. Both words mean "to expel potion," or antidote. An antidote is a medicine you take to keep a poison in your body from harming you.

Humans aren't the only ones with bezoars. It may sound bizarre, but bezoars found in animals were once thought to be magical medicine that could be used as an antidote.

In 1567, France's King Charles IX had a curious surgeon named Ambroise Paré. Dr. Paré wanted to test the bezoar's possible powers as a poison antidote. The tricky part was finding someone willing to take poison.

It so happened a cook in the king's household stole some fancy silverware and was sentenced to be hanged. (Yikes. A little harsh, King Chuck!) Since the cook had nothing to lose, he agreed to take the poison—*if* Dr. Paré gave him a "magic" bezoar with the poison, and *if* he was promised that *if* he lived, he would be set free.

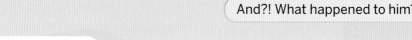

CHUCK: That's an *iffy* situation!

PROFESSOR ANITA PUKE: No ifs, ands, or buts about it.

And?! What happened to him?

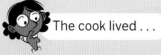

The cook lived . . .

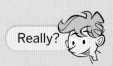

Really?

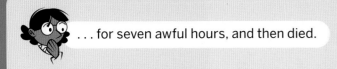
. . . for seven awful hours, and then died.

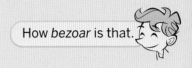
How *bezoar* is that.

Motion Sickness Before Modern Times

Prepare for a Barfy Ride

Flying on an airplane today could be compared to a bus ride. You take your seat, look out the window or read, and get out at your destination. While you're traveling in a plane's pressurized cabin (with clean air pumped in for safety and comfort) with a pilot who can fly at high altitudes above rough weather, you're likely to have a smooth ride.

But air travel used to mean sitting in a cabin filled with exhaust fumes, the sound of rumbling engines, and a frightfully bumpy ride. In 1911, this hair-raising air experience led French researchers René Cruchet and René Moulinier to diagnose a brand-new "disease"—airsickness.

Despite these challenges, airlines did their best to make passengers comfy. Some even hired nurses to join their flight crews to help passengers feel more secure. In the 1920s, paper airsickness bags were handed out, or even fancy china barf bowls.

QUEEZY: I would not want to do the dishes after those flights.

In the mid-1930s, some airlines offered gagging guests creative options for collecting belly jelly, like buckets made of papier-mâché (layers of paper and glue molded into a shape). But overall, people were becoming more comfortable with air travel. Improved planes helped, for sure. Researchers also think travelers having more experience in the air contributed to less airsickness. Maybe the more often passengers flew, the better the brain could adapt to the eye/brain mismatch of motion sickness.

**More trust in air travel + mental strength =
fewer worries and less airsickness**

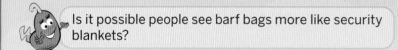

Is it possible people see barf bags more like security blankets?

Sounds like a safe assumption to me.

Meet the Barf Bag Inventor

The first plastic-lined "barf bag" was created by inventor Gilmore "Shelly" Schjeldahl for Bemis Bag Company. He sold his design to Northwest Orient Airlines in 1949.

Mr. Schjeldahl didn't stop there. After helping passengers in the air, he set his sights even higher. He went on to create large communication satellites for NASA that could revolve around the Earth every two hours.

Barf Bag Museum

Fact: People collect barf bags.

Obvious question: WHY?

Collectors of barf bags see them like a souvenir. You know, like bringing home a snowglobe or a seashell to remind you of your trip.

The caretaker of an online airsickness bag museum stores his "souvenirs" in protective plastic sheets snapped into binders. (Wouldn't want barf bags to get messy, right?)

Guinness World Records reports that as of February 2012, Niek Vermeulen of the Netherlands owned 6,290 (unused!) airsickness bags. People who trade barf bags or donate them to collectors are called Patrons of Puke.

 Almost sounds like rock collecting, doesn't it? But not.

Did You Know?

In April 2023, singer and songwriter Dolly Parton told a National Public Radio host that she keeps a little tape recorder or notepad with her so she's ready if she gets an idea for a new song. But if she's on a plane, she just writes it on a barf bag!

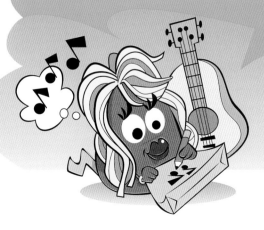

QUEEZY: I could help Ms. Parton write a beautiful barf bag ballad.

Barfday Cake

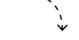

MAKES 8 SERVINGS

YOU WILL NEED:

• 1 premade angel food cake (the kind with a hole in the center)

Cake-hole filling

• 2 cups vanilla pudding (use premade or make from a mix)
• Chunky bits to mix into pudding—broken cookies, cut-up gummy worms, chopped nuts, raisins or dried cranberries, chocolate chips, crisp rice cereal

Cake glaze

• 2 cups confectioners sugar (it's the powdery white sugar)
• Milk or water
• Food coloring—1 drop red and yellow (to make orange)
• ¼ cup raisins
• ¼ cup graham cracker crumbs

⭐ **Before you begin:** Practice food safety (and avoid the vomit). Always start by washing your hands and cleaning the area of the kitchen where you'll be cooking. You'll want an adult to help you. Make sure your assistant has clean hands too!

HERE'S WHAT YOU NEED TO DO:

Step 1: Put the cake in a big bowl (or a clean bucket!).

Step 2: In a separate bowl, mix vanilla pudding with your favorite chunky bits. (Don't use too many chunks. You want the filling to stay gooey.)

Step 3: Spoon filling into the center of the cake.

Step 4: Make the cake glaze.

• Put 2 cups of powdered sugar in a bowl.

• Add 2 tablespoons of water or milk to sugar and stir or whisk.

• Add a little more milk/water as needed until the glaze is smooth and runny enough to pour off the mixing spoon.

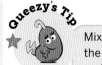

Queezy's Tip

Mix Puke Punch to go with the Barfday Cake. Find the recipe on page 161.

• Add 1 drop each of red and yellow food coloring, and sprinkle in a handful of raisins. Mix again.

Step 5: Drizzle the glaze over the cake. Sprinkle on graham cracker crumbs while the glaze is still wet.

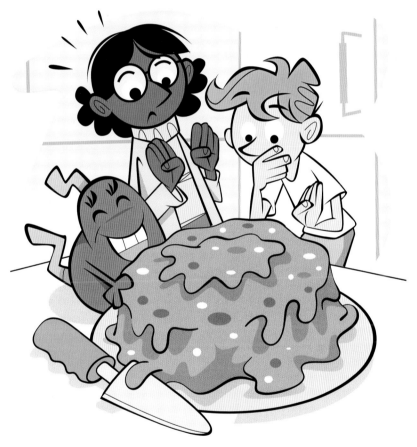

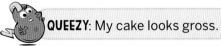

QUEEZY: My cake looks gross.

CHUCK: Congratulations! You did it right!

25

Barfday Party Barf Bag

```
`- - - ->` MAKES ONE BAG
```

This bag filled with puke party favors may help when your friends feel nauseous or need to barf. (Let's hope it's not during your party!)

Queezy's Tip

Suggestion: Keep this barf bag in your backpack "just in case"!

YOU WILL NEED:

• 2 paper lunch bags for each party guest

• Markers

• Party favors (see ideas below)

Barf Bag Bonus! Get extra gross and add an MYO "gag gift." For more gross-piration, see page 77.

HERE'S WHAT YOU NEED TO DO:

Step 1: Draw a label on the bag. Come up with your own label or use one of these ideas:

• MY Barf Bag—Get Your Own!

• Barf-uh-teria Special

• Barf Bag—Open at your own risk!

• _____'s Gag Bag
(Write your friend's name.)

Step 2: Open the bag with the label and slip the other (unopened) bag inside, and then open it so one bag fits inside the other. This will help the bag hold heavier party favors, like bottled water. And the extra bag may come in handy in case of you know what!

Step 3: Fill bag with pukey party favors, like these:

• Breath mints or gum

• Small bottle of water

• Crackers

• Tissues

• Hand wipes

• A funny photo or joke—something to make your friend smile!

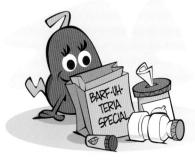

*Bumba is known as a creator god to the
Kuba people of the Democratic Republic of the Congo in Central Africa.*

Bumba Barfs the World

Before the world began, there was only darkness, water, and Bumba, the first ancestor of all. Alone in the damp darkness, Bumba vomited Sun with her brilliant light. Sun's warmth dried the water, and outlines of land could be seen.

Exhilarated by his own imagination, Bumba vomited up radiant Moon and dazzling stars. But he wasn't done yet!

Bumba vomited once again, and amazing creatures appeared: a leopard, a crested eagle, a crocodile, a fish, a tortoise, a heron, a beetle, and a goat. Oh! And from a flourish of Bumba's vomit came Lightning as well. As his grand finale, Bumba vomited many humans.

Inspired by Bumba, the animals created too. The fish fashioned all varieties of fish, and the beetle produced all other insects. In a surprising twist, the crocodile created snakes and the Iguana. Astounding work! Yet there was more to do.

Enter the three sons of Bumba, ready to finish the world. First son Nyonye Ngana tried to make white ants, but he died trying. Second son Chonganda created a plant from which all trees and plants sprung. Third son Chedi Bumba chose to go in a different direction by creating a bird of prey known as a kite.

Meanwhile, Lightning became such a bother, Bumba chased her into the sky. Relentless Lightning kept striking the earth, so Bumba returned his attention to humans. He revealed the secret that every tree contains fire and showed the humans how to bring that fire out for nighttime warmth and light.

Imagine that! Starting with only darkness and water, Bumba, the first ancestor of all, hurled a world of wonders.

CHUCK'S SICK SCIENCE

Black Holes Barf Star Bits

In space, no one can hear you slurp.

In 2016, scientists observed a supermassive black hole 308 million light-years from Earth. It was in elliptical galaxy NGC 4889 at the center of a giant cluster of 2,000 galaxies. (Talk about a crowded neighborhood!)

Now, get this—that colossal black hole (21 billion times the mass of Earth's sun) "spaghettified" a star by pulling and stretching it before swallowing the star whole. That's right—a black hole made "star pasta." Then, in a burst of light, the black hole spewed star specks into space!

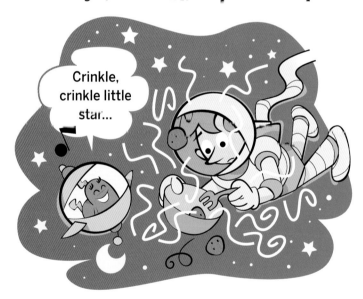

Crinkle, crinkle little star...

EVER HEARD OF THE VOMIT COMET?

Orbit over to page 223 for more space-sick stuff.

BIOHAZARD! THIS IS A "NO TOUCHY" SUBJECT

A biohazard is a virus, bacteria, or fungus that can harm humans or other living things. Fluids like vomit, blood, and urine are biohazards because they may contain diseases. That's why it's important to wear gloves when cleaning up someone else's vomit and to wash your hands after.

A special product made of an absorbent gel powder can be used to soak up vomit quickly. The powder contains a disinfectant to help kill germs and prevent them from spreading. Once the powder dries, it can be scraped up and thrown away safely.

BRACE YOURSELF

What Do You Do if You BWWB (Barf While Wearing Braces)?

If you BWWB, do *not* rush to brush or make haste with that toothpaste. As tough as it is, wait at least thirty minutes before you brush.

Why wait? Barfing brings up stomach acid (along with other "stuff"). Acid clings to the inside of your mouth post-puke. If you brush right after you make yuck, you'll be

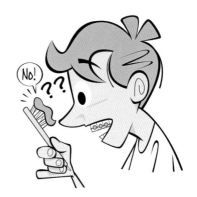

spreading that acid around. Besides brushing acid into your teeth, you may even move it to parts of your mouth the acid wouldn't have reached without your help.

Until it's safe to brush, you can rinse out your mouth with water or swish around antiseptic mouthwash. Or you could mix 1 teaspoon of baking soda into a glass of warm water, take a sip, swoosh it around your mouth, and spit. Bonus: It will help freshen your breath too!

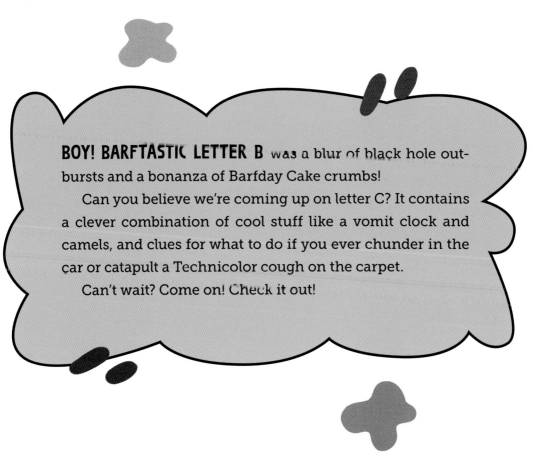

BOY! BARFTASTIC LETTER B was a blur of black hole outbursts and a bonanza of Barfday Cake crumbs!

Can you believe we're coming up on letter C? It contains a clever combination of cool stuff like a vomit clock and camels, and clues for what to do if you ever chunder in the car or catapult a Technicolor cough on the carpet.

Can't wait? Come on! Check it out!

C

Congratulations! Letter C is crowded with chunk-tastic content like **Chuck's Coloring Book of Chunk** (crayons not required).

Care to guess what **car sickness, cybersickness,** and **camel sickness** have in common? Catch the secret to **cleaning up carpet collywobbles** too. Craving crunchy crab cakes or creamy clam chowder? Careful! It could all be **contaminated**!

TURN UP THE VOLUME ON YOUR
VOMIT VOCABULARY

Calling Ralph: call up an ice cream cone on the porcelain phone

Carpet the Grass: make a chuck yawn and feed the lawn

Cascade the Cat: spew kitten chow

Chew Backward: pizza goes in (chew-chew-chew), pizza comes out (ew-ew-ew)

Chew the Cheese: hurl an absurd pile of curds

Chuck: toss the anchovy pizza sauce

Chuckle on the Bus: the meals in the gut go round and round

Chum Bucket: *see* fish salad swish

Chunder: the rumble of thunder down under before the brekky (Aussie for breakfast) rains into the dunny (toilet)

Chunk: dunk a pukey hunk that stinks like a skunk

Clean House: plop stomach slop, stop, and then mop

Collywobbles: nervous tummy rumbles followed by a chunder storm

CHUCK'S SICK SCIENCE

C Is for Contamination

PROFESSOR ANITA PUKE: Whether your family picks up dinner at a deli, orders takeout from a restaurant, or makes meals at home, sometimes food can be unsafe to eat if bacteria have contaminated it. Bacteria may be tiny, but they can cause *big* problems when they multiply inside the body.

CHUCK: Bacteria multiply? Can they add and subtract too?

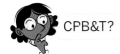
Focus, Chuck. Bacteria can give you infections that cause fever, cramps, and—you guessed it—vomiting.

And that's why I can never look at a CPB&T sandwich again.

CPB&T?

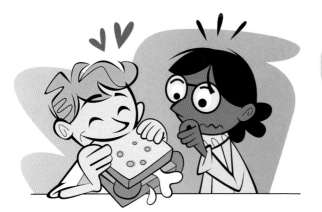

You know, chunky peanut butter and tuna.

Thank you, Chuck. Now *I* feel sick.

Queezy's Question

Can I tell if my burrito is—*gulp*—contaminated?

 PROFESSOR ANITA PUKE: Bacteria are so small, you cannot see, taste, or smell them.

QUEEZY: Or hear them?

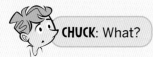 **CHUCK**: What?

We're doomed. *Gulp. Gulp.*

 Hey, not *all* bacteria are bad, remember?

Phew!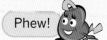

 But if certain kinds of bad bacteria end up in your food, they can make you sick. That's called food poisoning. For example, some types of the bacteria *E. coli* can cause diarrhea, stomach cramps, or vomiting if they're in food or drinking water

To quote a genius, "We're doomed."

 There are ways to protect yourself.

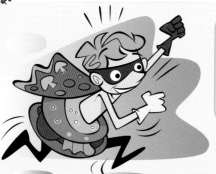 Never fear! Super Chuck is here! Protector of pizza! Guardian of garbanzo beans! Champion of cheese! Defender of dumplings! Preserver of parsnips! Keeper of kiwi! Bodyguard of baklava! Rescuer of roast beef!

 Hmm. We're doomed.

BE THE PROTECTOR against food poisoning at your house. Go to page 106.

CHUCK'S SICK SCIENCE

Cybersickness

Don't scroll past this one!

 CHUCK: I asked Professor Anita Puke for this info "just in case" Queezy and I ever play video games.

QUEEZY: Have you ever been

scrolling,

scrolling,

scrolling

on your computer or phone when—uh-oh—suddenly you feel dizzy or even nauseous?

You may have a form of motion sickness called cybersickness.

Cybersickness may also make you feel like the room is spinning. If you're on a computer or gaming in a stinky or stuffy room, cybersickness may even cause you to "clean house" (as in, hurl!).

Cybersickness Is a Matter of Mixed Messages

Let's say you're wearing a virtual reality (VR) headset to play a 3D game that simulates movement through the headset.

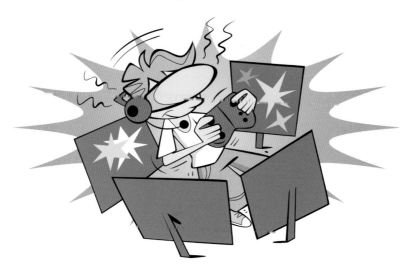

The eyes tell the brain: "Whoa! We're gliding up, down, and around a mountain on the back of a barb-tailed dragon!"

The vestibular system (aka the inner ear that senses movement and balance) says: "Head level, looking ahead, steady as she goes."

And then the proprioceptive system (located in your joints and muscles, allowing you to sense movement, tension, and pressure) chimes in: "Nope. Nothing new to sense here."

These confusing messages can give you a weird "Where am I?" sensation. You may feel nauseous, especially if you just ate a big meal or you already feel "under the weather."

How to Combat Cybersickness

• Get up, stretch, and grab a light snack to avoid playing on an empty tank.

- Give your eyes a timeout. Look away from the screen regularly, and focus on something that's not moving.

- Use one screen at a time instead of looking at the computer, glancing at the TV, and checking your phone all at once. Slow the scroll.

If you start to feel dizzy or nauseated during screen time:

- Stand slowly. Step away from the TV or close the laptop. Stretch.

- Take deep breaths and exhale slowly.

- Open a window or use a fan to keep air moving. (Stuffy rooms make nausea worse.)

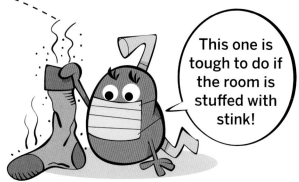

This one is tough to do if the room is stuffed with stink!

FOR MORE on other kinds of motion sickness, fly over to page 21.

FIND THE INSIDE SCOOP on the inner ear and balance. Head over to page 17. (Take your time. Watch your step. Don't trip.)

FOR A FORECAST ON where the expression "under the weather" came from, sail on over to page 213.

CAR SICKNESS 101

Yield for Vehicular Vomit

If your plan to steer clear of car sickness goes out the window, do your best to put the brakes on the bleh with these tips, like making a Hurl Hammock!

- Keep a plastic bag in your backpack that you can use, tie up, and toss.

- Ask the driver to pull over so you can chunder outside the car. If you can safely leave the vehicle to unload on the grass, dirt, asphalt, or anywhere other than the car you must get back into, give it a go.

- If getting out of the vehicle is not an option (maybe you're on a highway, it's pouring rain, zombie bears are lumbering just outside, etc.), ask the driver if they can safely pull over so you can chew the cheese and splatter the sploshy mouth sneeze right out the window. The car will need a wash later, but better outside than in! (Do not stick your head out the window of a moving vehicle!)

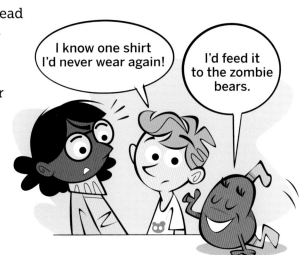

I know one shirt I'd never wear again!

I'd feed it to the zombie bears.

- If there's nothing in the car to make collywobbles into, you may need to vomit on yourself. Grab your shirt and pull it up around your mouth to make a hammock for your hurl. Yes, that's the nightmare scenario. It's still better than heaving a pile of stinky vomit into your friend's backseat. (But if you do—hey, it happens to lots of people!—see Uncle Urp's 5½ Tips for Cleaning Up Carpet Collywobbles.)

UNCLE URP'S 5½ TIPS FOR CLEANING UP CARPET COLLYWOBBLES

What you wish you didn't need to know but will be glad you do . . .

Act fast! Keep chunder from seeping down under (as in sinking into the carpet). Pull on gloves before you start.

Step 1: Scrape off any wet sloppy stuff with a spoon or piece of stiff cardboard.

Step 2: Sprinkle baking soda over the crime scene to soak up the upchuck and deal with the stink.

Step 3: Let the baking soda sit for up to 30 minutes, then vacuum it up.

Step 4: Fluff the carpet with your fingers. (See? Gloves were a good idea!)

Step 5: Smell your fingers. Are they fresh or funky? If a foul odor is still there, spray the spot with pet stain remover and follow the directions on the bottle.

Step 5½: Try to never "carpet the grass" on carpeting ever again (if you can help it).

IT'S CLOCK TIME

Two Words: Vomit Clock!

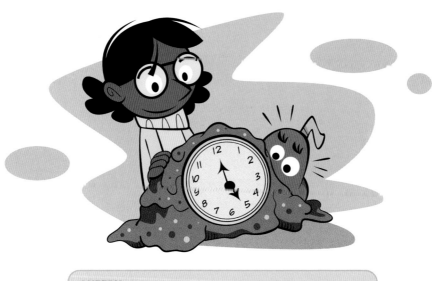

QUEEZY: It's your first *time* hearing about a vomit clock? Take a *second* to read this and try not to be *alarmed*.

According to the Vomit Clock Museum, do-it-yourself clock craft kits were popular from about 1950 to 1970. (No one called them vomit clocks back then.) These kits contained small stones, glitter, dried plants, shells, and colored glass to drop into a clock-shaped mold filled with liquid resin. (It looks like thick clear glue.) Once the resin hardened, the mold was removed to reveal a handmade clock with the little objects suspended in it.

Years later, in 2018, a Facebook thrift store group posted the term "vomit clock." With the look of odd objects floating in clear goo, it's not hard to see how the clocks got that nickname.

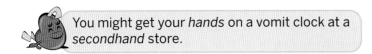
You might get your *hands* on a vomit clock at a *secondhand* store.

CHUCK: Where do you come up with all these wisecracks?

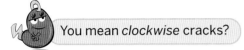
You mean *clockwise* cracks?

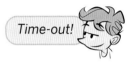
Time-out!

CHUCK'S COLORING BOOK OF CHUNK

Please "color" inside the lines!

Obscene Green

Ever wonder why your vomit might look greenish yellow? More than likely, bile is to blame. The liver makes bile, stores it in the gallbladder, and then sends it to the stomach to help process the incoming food, which in your case just became takeout.

Barfy Brown

But what if the vomit looks a little more like mud? Brown food is most likely the reason for *that* color of vomit. Maybe you poked too much chocolate pudding down the shoot? It's not common in kids, but another reason for brown, root-beer-like color is bleeding in the stomach. If that happens, tell an adult. You may need to go to a doctor to make sure you're okay.

Clear Cascade

Hurling clear fluid is normal, especially if you've already vomited the chunky stuff, or if you have a stomach bug or you're vomiting on an empty gut. Clear spew may also happen if you drink a lot of water too quickly and your stomach can't handle the overload.

Weird White

If you happen to guzzle a glass of milk or chow an ice cream cone or crunch cauliflower with veggie dip right before you chunder, you may make a weird white puddle. The vomit may look foamy, especially if you have a gassy gut when you clean house.

Puke Pink or Red

Bright red blood in the vomit may be due to swallowing blood from a bloody nose, a cut lip, a sore spot from your braces, or even pulling out a loose tooth. If there's just a bit of blood and it doesn't keep coming up, it's probably not a big deal. Sometimes bloody vomit happens if the body has trouble digesting milk products. An adult—and a doctor, if needed—can help you sort things out.

Out of the Blue Barf

Barfing up blue is very rare. It's caused by accidentally swallowing a poison used to kill ants or roaches or a toxic chemical used to kill weeds. Be careful to never, ever drink these products!

ORANGE PUKE? See page 153 for "Oh! Orange Vomit!"

LEARN MORE ABOUT BILE
by sliding on over to page 5.

CHUCK'S SICK SCIENCE

It's About Chyme!

PROFESSOR ANITA PUKE: *Chyme* is pronounced *kime.* It rhymes with *time.* (And no, it's not related to vomit clocks.) The word *chyme* is from a Greek word that means "juice." Chyme is a mushy mix of partly digested food, stomach acid, digestive enzymes, and gastric juices. The stomach pushes chyme through the pyloric valve and into the duodenum [doo-uh-DEE-num].

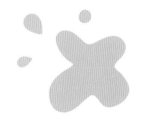

CHUCK: Excuse me. Pie lick what? The duo who-oh?

The pyloric valve is located at the lower end of the stomach. It's in charge of letting the partly processed food leave the stomach and head into the duodenum. The duodenum is the start of the small intestine.

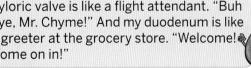

QUEEZY: Oooh! I have to chime in! My pyloric valve is like a flight attendant. "Buh bye, Mr. Chyme!" And my duodenum is like a greeter at the grocery store. "Welcome! Come on in!"

HURLED HISTORY

Oh, C'mon. Camel Sickness?

When General Napoléon Bonaparte of France led his first military campaign against Egypt in 1798, he created a "camel corps." Camels are known as the "ships of the desert." Since two thirds of Egypt is desert, camels made a lot more sense than riding horses into battle.

Napoléon discovered the downside of the up-and-down and side-to-side motion of camel-riding—it made him nauseous. But Napoleon rode one anyway. And he came to appreciate his camel so much that when it finally died of old age, it was preserved and displayed in a museum.

His soldiers who overcame motion sickness still had to get off their camels to shoot (unlike firing a rifle on horseback). So, not ideal. Some soldiers were useless because they couldn't conquer the sand/sea camel sickness in a land where every day was Hump Day.

QUEEZY: I bet they said, "We can't *sand* this!" But in French, of course.

THE LETTER D dares you to dive into the digestive system, along with the wet and dry sides of vomit, plus more of Queezy's inquisitive questions. There's a disgusting-looking delicious snack recipe waiting for you too.

Let's take a dip!

D

Deep breathing is recommended before diving into details on **dehydration** and **dry heaving.** Dreaming of a snack? There's a Ralph-worthy Recipe for **Dry Heave Dip** waiting for you to digest.

Dare you to dig in!

TURN UP THE VOLUME ON YOUR VOMIT VOCABULARY

Decorate the Doorknob: splatter the door, then three times more

Deliver Groceries: bag eggs, bread, and milk in the belly—then drop them at the bathroom door

Dinner to Go: when you dine and the dinner dashes

Download Dinner: transfer the bile file to "commode overflowed" code

Drive the Porcelain Bus: grab the toilet-seat-shaped steering wheel while the bus is unloading

Drown Your Desk: sit in science class and see a notebook swimming in gut goop

Dry Heave: honk hot air as you stare at the toilet down there

Dunk: drop damp doughnuts, as in "Hey, Queezy, downing a dozen jelly doughnuts after soccer will make me dunk!"

CHUCK'S SICK SCIENCE

D Is for Digestive System

The digestive system includes body parts like the mouth, throat, belly, and intestines, which work when you eat or drink.

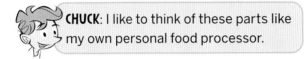

CHUCK: I like to think of these parts like my own personal food processor.

The digestive system's job is to soak up the nutrients and water from the food you eat. Then it says heave-ho to things your body doesn't need.

Insider Intelligence on Your Digestive System

Want to know something far-out? The human body has no problem swallowing or digesting food in zero gravity. That means munching a meal in outer space works about the same as eating on Earth.

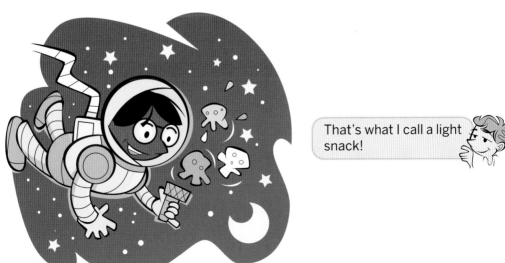

That's what I call a light snack!

DEHYDRATION

Your body is about 60 percent fluid. Throwing up over and over can cause your body to lose a lot of the water you need to be healthy. That's called being dehydrated.

Dehydration Needs Rehydration

When replacing fluid you lose from vomiting, sip slowly. Drinking too much too fast can upset your stomach again. These are good choices for helping you rehydrate and have less nausea:

- Herbal tea, such as chamomile, peppermint, ginger, or green tea (with a little sugar, honey, or agave for sweetener, if you like)

- Water (room temperature or cold)

- Sports drinks with electrolytes to give your body back the calcium, sodium, and potassium it needs

- Freezer pops

- Apple juice

- Gelatin

- Clear broth

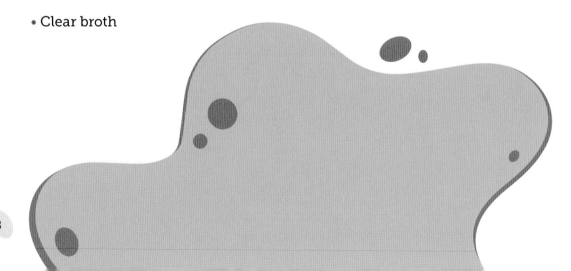

DEEP BREATHING

For stress relieving when you feel like heaving:

- Take in a deep breath through your nose to fill your lungs.

- Feel your belly get bigger as you take in the air.

- Let the air out slowly through your mouth or nose.

- Let your belly relax.

- Repeat.

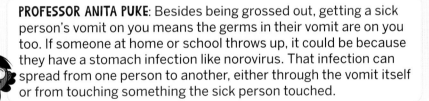

Queezy's Question

Disinfect that doorknob? Ew! What happens if somebody's barf gets on me?

PROFESSOR ANITA PUKE: Besides being grossed out, getting a sick person's vomit on you means the germs in their vomit are on you too. If someone at home or school throws up, it could be because they have a stomach infection like norovirus. That infection can spread from one person to another, either through the vomit itself or from touching something the sick person touched.

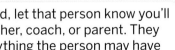

QUEEZY: Sounds like a touchy subject.

If you see that someone has vomited, let that person know you'll get help. Tell an adult, like your teacher, coach, or parent. They can cover the vomit and clean everything the person may have touched. This will help to prevent the spread of germs.

Dry Heave Dip

MAKES 4 SERVINGS

YOU WILL NEED:

- 15 oz. jar salsa con queso
- 15 oz. jar salsa
- ½ cup refried beans
- 1 cup sour cream
- Optional chunky add-ins: sliced black olives, canned corn (with water drained), chopped tomato, chopped green onion
- Dry, salty, crunchy tortilla chips

Before you begin: Practice food safety (and avoid the vomit). Always start by washing your hands and cleaning the area of the kitchen where you'll be cooking. You'll want an adult to help you. Make sure your assistant has clean hands too!

HERE'S WHAT YOU NEED TO DO:

Step 1. Mix the ingredients (minus the chips) in a serving bowl. If you're not going to eat the dip right away, put it in the refrigerator.

Step 2: Serve the dip with a bowl of tortilla chips. Do not leave the dip out for more than one hour. Keep leftovers in a covered container in the refrigerator.

DONE DIGESTING LETTER D? Do some deep breathing to decompress (even if you don't feel sick) and grab some a favorite drink to stay hydrated. As you exit letter D, don't forget to disinfect the doorknob on the way out!

Eager to enter letter E? Even more earpy entries and erupting grocery geysers are everywhere! And educate yourself on the meaning of one of Professor Puke's favorite words—*emesis.*

E

Ever wonder if there's an easier way to say "**erupting grocery geyser**"? Evidently there is. Explore an excellent explanation of the **epiglottis.** And not to make you uneasy, but we'll even examine the **enteric nervous system.** There's also an **egg**-ceptional Ralph-worthy Recipe to enjoy.

TURN UP THE VOLUME ON YOUR VOMIT VOCABULARY

Earp: swiftly slurp, then burp and blow

Eat Backward: chew through a ton of cashews and then they come back to you

Elevator: send lunch for a ride from the belly floor to the top floor

Emergency Stomach Evacuation: when the stomach calls "Everybody exit!"

Emesis Me: dribble barf down the belly

Erupting Grocery Geyser: eat every treat from the store before the gut tosses them back in the bag

Exit Emesis: direct the snack to the nearest exit

CHUCK'S SICK SCIENCE

Whether you prefer to call it earping, erupting, or eating backward, if you really want to impress your science teacher, check out this en-*gross*-ing medical term.

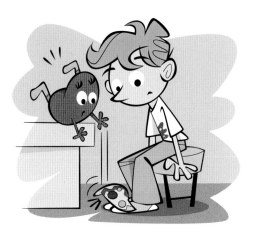 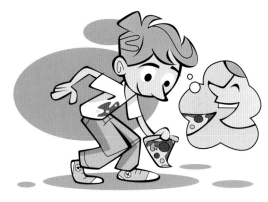

E Is for Emesis

Emesis is a medical term that comes from a Greek word *emein*. It's pronounced EH-muh-suss.

 CHUCK: Tell me if I got this right. Emesis is the fancy-pants, proper term for eating backward.

PROESSOR ANITA PUKE: To be precise, emesis is the oral eviction of gastrointestinal contents, due to contractions of the gut and the muscles of the thoracoabdominal wall.

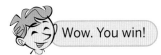 Wow. You win!

And you win too. Emesis can mean eating backward. (And it's easier to say!)

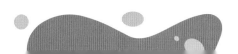

EPIGLOTTIS

Put a Lid on It

The epiglottis is a small cartilage "lid" located at the base of the tongue toward the very back of the throat. Cartilage is tough, flexible tissue. (It's what gives your ears and nose their shape too.) The epiglottis folds back to keep what you eat or drink from sliding down the windpipe when you swallow. Once you've swallowed, the "lid" goes back to an upright position so that air can enter the larynx (voice box) and lungs.

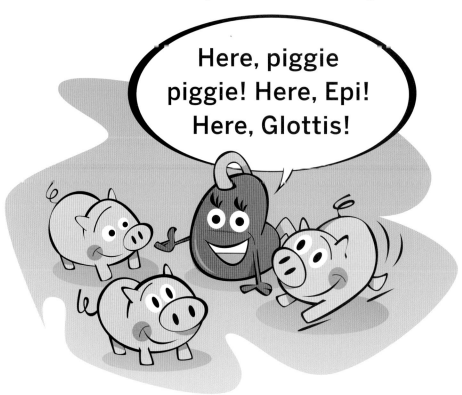

Here, piggie piggie! Here, Epi! Here, Glottis!

QUEEZY: Now I get it! I thought it was "e-*pig*-lottis," a fancy-pants Latin word for a lot of pigs.

ENTERIC NERVOUS SYSTEM

Because Two Brains Are Better Than One

You've heard of the central nervous system (CNS). It has two parts: the brain and the spinal cord. But have you met the enteric nervous system (ENS)? The ENS works with the CNS, but it can do some jobs on its own too.

The enteric nervous system is huge. We're talking 600 million neurons! It goes from the esophagus (the part that connects the throat and the stomach) through the stomach and intestines and down to the anus (the very end of the large intestine where poop comes out). Among other things, this system coordinates the process of digestion and makes it possible for the body to absorb nutrients.

Scientists are learning more about the enteric nervous system and its connection to the rest of the body—including the way it "talks" to the brain. The enteric nervous system is even called a second brain (located in the gut instead of the head).

QUEEZY: I had a gut feeling about this. And I always listen to my gut. It has such a cute voice.

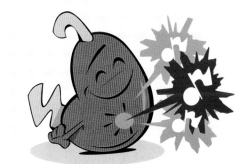

DID YOU HEAR THAT?
EAR INFECTIONS CAUSE EARP

An ear infection is caused by a buildup of fluid in the ear. This can make you feel like you have motion sickness. Your balance may be off. You may be dizzy or feel nauseous and end up vomiting.

CHUCK: I need to hear somebody say I can't vomit out my ears.

QUEEZY: That sounds like an ear-rational thing to worry about.

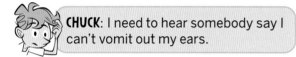

Queezy's Question

My friend Fizzy is afraid to "eat backward." Is there a name for that?

PROFESSOR ANITA PUKE: A person who is afraid to vomit has emetophobia—fear of emesis. Needing to throw up or seeing someone else vomit can make the fear even worse.

QUEEZY: Poor Fizzy.

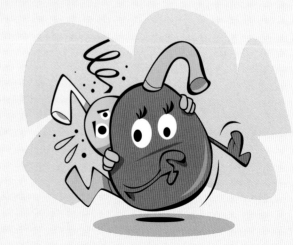

Earps in a Basket

This recipe puts a tummy twist on "eggs in a basket."

MAKES 2 SERVINGS

 Before you begin: Practice food safety (and avoid the vomit). Always start by washing your hands and cleaning the area of the kitchen where you'll be cooking. You'll want an adult to help you. Make sure your assistant has clean hands too!

YOU WILL NEED:

* 2 eggs
* 2 pieces of bread
* 2 tablespoons soft butter
* Salt and pepper
* Green and yellow food coloring

HERE'S WHAT YOU NEED TO DO:

Step 1: Put bread in toaster. While it's toasting . . .

Step 2: Crack eggs into a bowl, add food coloring, and use a whisk or fork to mix well.

Step 3: In a small frying pan, melt a pat of butter over medium-low heat.

Step 4: Pour in the egg mixture. Push it around in the pan with a spatula to scramble.

Step 5: Butter the toast and put it on plates.

Step 6: Press a glass or round cookie cutter into the center of the toast. Lift out the toast's "belly" and save it.

Step 7: Scoop eggs into each toast hole. Salt and pepper. Top with a toast belly to surprise someone who's not egg-specting earps under there!

Queezy's Question

Ka-choo! I can't keep my eyes open when I sneeze. Can I have an erupting grocery geyser with my eyes open?

 PROFESSOR ANITA PUKE: Yes, you can vomit with open eyes (if you like to see your lunch *again*!).

 QUEEZY: You're sure my eyes won't pop out?

 No eye popping. Promise. But you may want to close your eyes anyway . . . for comfort, at the very least.

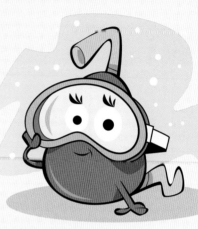

EARS, EYES, AND AN EPIGLOTTIS—everybody has them, but not everyone knows what you know about them. Not even close!

Next up, the letter F. Spoiler alert—the F stands for *fun*. Well, not the part about food poisoning . . . but you *will* find instructions for a fake chunky puddle for fooling your friends!

Farewell, letter E! Fast-forward to fascinating letter F!

F

For starters, you'll find **face fountain** folklore from Tibet, followed by facts about **food poisoning.** Feel free to follow a frosty recipe for **Frozen Frothy Cough Pops.** There's a for-real recipe for **fake vomit** too. No fooling!

TURN UP THE VOLUME ON YOUR VOMIT VOCABULARY

Face Fountain: feel pink lemonade and orange soda flow down your frown

Fast Food: when you see (and feel) your sausage sandwich speed away

Feed the Fishes: let the minnows munch your pro-munched lunch

Flash: when your dinner decides to dash

Flounder: when your stomach flips and your fish dinner flops

Food Fire Drill: eat spicy rice and feel it head for the emergency exit

Forge Ahead: where mashed potatoes meet water gravy

Free Soup: when your misery makes a big bowl of mystery

Frothy Cough: foam root beer float from your face

FAKE VOMIT— HOLLYWOOD-STYLE HURL

Visual effects artists are quite the chefs of face fountain filler. If the script calls for it, these artisans of arf can whip up vast vats of barf (as in gallons!). They may use split pea soup, tomato paste, and frozen berries. Uncooked ramen noodles are used for texture. Yum.

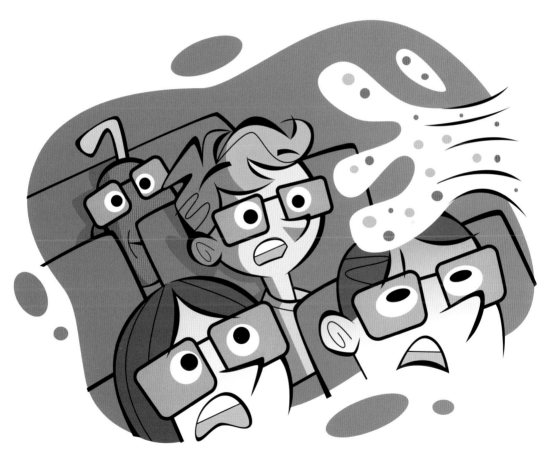

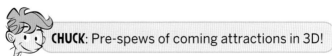

CHUCK: Pre-spews of coming attractions in 3D!

Fake Chunky Puddle

MAKES 1 INEDIBLE PUDDLE

YOU CAN START WITH THESE BASICS, BUT HAVE FUN CUSTOMIZING YOUR CHUNKY CONCOCTION:

- ¼ cup chunky applesauce or canned pumpkin
- 2 packets unflavored gelatin (from a 1 oz. box)
- Dry oatmeal, bran flakes, toaster crumbs, or ground graham crackers
- Rice, raisins, or uncooked ramen noodles

Before you begin: Practice food safety (and avoid the vomit). Always start by washing your hands and cleaning the area of the kitchen where you'll be cooking. You'll want an adult to help you. Make sure your assistant has clean hands too!

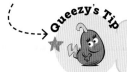

Queezy's Tip

This recipe is for fun, not food, but practicing food safety is always a good idea.

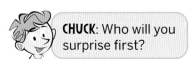

CHUCK: Who will you surprise first?

HERE'S WHAT YOU NEED TO DO:

Step 1: Pour the applesauce or pumpkin into a nonstick frying pan. Warm it over low heat.

Step 2: Stir in the unflavored gelatin.

Step 3: Mix in a pinch of oatmeal and the flakes/crumbs or ground crackers. Use a spatula to form the curvy edges of the puddle.

Step 4: Remove from the heat. Sprinkle the bran flakes over the applesauce mixture or add a pinch of rice, raisins, or dry ramen noodles, if you like. Use your imagination!

Step 5: Allow the barf to cool before sliding it onto a plate with a spatula.

F IS FOR FOOD POISONING

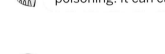 **PROFESSOR ANITA PUKE**: Meat, raw veggies, dairy products (milk, cheese, yogurt), seafood (oysters, shrimp, fish), bean sprouts, and eggs can be healthy and delicious. But if these foods are not stored, prepared, or cooked safely, and you eat them, germs or bacteria in the food can end up in your body. Becoming sick from contaminated food is called food poisoning. It can cause you to—

QUEEZY: Make "free soup"!

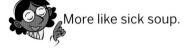 More like sick soup.

FUNNY TOP 200

In 2018, psychologist Chris Westbury with the University of Alberta in Canada conducted a study of 45,000 words in the English language. Out of all those words, Dr. Westbury came up with a list of the 200 words people find funniest. These words made the list:

Upchuck

Barfed

Puke

Pukes

Puking

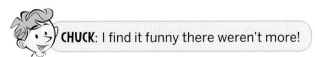 **CHUCK**: I find it funny there weren't more!

Queezy's Question

Can fear make me "feed the fish"?

PROFESSOR ANITA PUKE: The mind and the gut have a close connection. They may have two different jobs, but the nerves and the chemical sensors they share keep them "talking" to each other. Scientists call that the gut brain axis. It makes sense, then, that if the mind is feeling scared and nervous—maybe you're worried about moving to a new school or scared of flying in a plane for the first time—your gut may change the way you process food. You could get an upset stomach or feel nauseous. If you (like lots of kids) get anxious on opening night of your school play or before your gymnastics competition, you may . . .

QUEEZY: Feed the fishes!

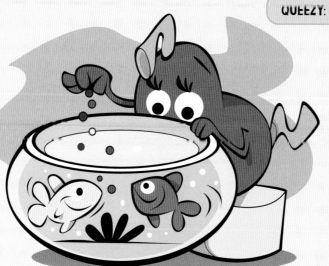

FIND OUT HOW to relieve stress
on page 179.

Frozen Frothy Cough Pops

MAKES 4 SERVINGS

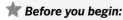 ***Before you begin:***
Practice food safety (and avoid the vomit). Always start by washing your hands and cleaning the area of the kitchen where you'll be cooking. You'll want an adult to help you. Make sure your assistant has clean hands too!

YOU WILL NEED:

- 4 cups orange juice (the more pulp, the better)
- ¾ cup vanilla yogurt
- 4 9 oz. disposable cups
- 1 gallon-size resealable plastic bag
- Wax paper or plastic wrap
- Aluminum foil
- Craft sticks

HERE'S WHAT YOU NEED TO DO:

Step 1: Put cups in a muffin tin (if you have one) to keep them from tipping over in the freezer.

Step 2: Pour juice and yogurt into a resealable plastic bag. Seal it tight and shake, shake, shake. Pour the "shake" into cups.

Step 3: Put plastic wrap or wax paper over the cups, then put a sheet of foil on top of that. Poke a craft stick into each cup. (Foil helps sticks stand up until the pops freeze. Wax paper or plastic wrap under the foil keeps the metal from reacting with acid in the juice.)

Step 4: Put the cups (still in the muffin tin) into the freezer. Check in about 30 minutes. If frozen, go to the next step.

Step 5: Peel or pull off outer cup. (If they stick, wrap your hands around the cup for 20 seconds and try again.)

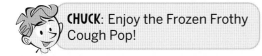 **CHUCK**: Enjoy the Frozen Frothy Cough Pop!

65

LETTER F never fails to fling fresh facts. How fun to find a recipe for a refreshing frothy treat to freeze for your friends.

Letter G grabs gobs of gross gargle gravy to make you grin and your imagination glow. Speaking of glow, you get to greet a growling lion who gurps gifts of gold—except for the greedy!

Let's *go*!

G

Greetings! Get the scoop on why gobbling raw cookie dough is a no-no. Engross yourself in a gory story of a **Greek god** who upchucked his children. See how gazing through special **glasses** can put the brakes on motion sickness. Get the creative juices flowing with instructions to make a groovy **gag gift.** There are gobs more gross stuff. Go get it!

TURN UP THE VOLUME ON YOUR VOMIT VOCABULARY

Gag: when you dry heave to relieve the zig-zag-do-I-need-a-barf-bag nag in the gut

Gargle Gravy: pack away mashed potatoes, then spew your spuds

Goodbye Pie: feel flaky before the crusty dessert deserts you

Goop: ploop out soggy soup

Gunk: what you hurl from the trunk

Gurp: belch up a spinach smoothie

Gush: hurl slush and rush to flush

Gut Grief: when you wolf down a sidewalk pizza (or six) and a whole Barfday Cake

Gut Soup: spew stomach slop with crumbled crackers

CHUCK'S SICK SCIENCE

Gastroparesis

Gastroparesis is a condition that keeps the belly from working right. The stomach muscles are supposed to squeeze and flex to create a wavelike action that causes the food in the gut to move down the digestive tract.

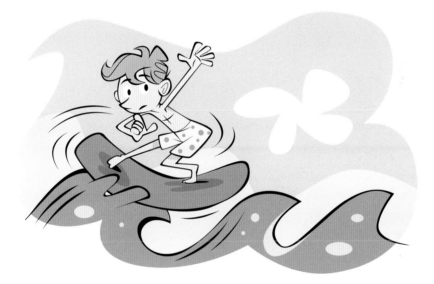

With gastroparesis, the muscles needed to make a wave action are too weak to move the partly digested food and chyme from the stomach to the small intestine. Signs of gastroparesis include nausea and vomiting, especially of undigested food.

SPEND A LITTLE TIME
learning about chyme on page 43.

GLASSES FOR MOTION SICKNESS? YOU MUST SEE THIS!

Motion sickness glasses have two round lenses on the front, just like you'd expect. But then there's a round lens for both sides of the head too. Lenses are filled with a blue liquid around the rim. The idea is that the liquid will move as the boat/car/plane moves, and that will trick the brain into thinking everything is in balance, and that means no motion sickness.

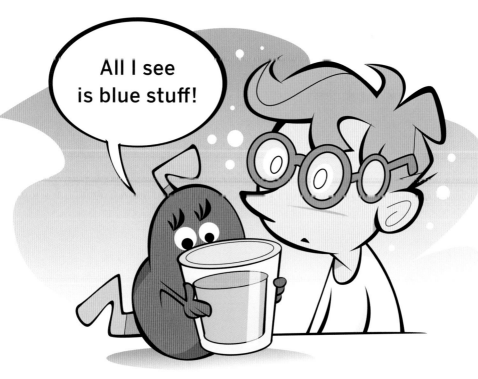

NEED TO KNOW MORE about the ups and downs
of motion sickness? Go to page 126.

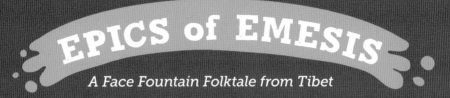

A Face Fountain Folktale from Tibet

The Gold-Vomiting Lion

There once was a family with a father, a mother, and two grown sons. After the father died, the brothers continued to live with their mother in a big house situated in a beautiful valley. The older brother was smart but also coldhearted and selfish, while the younger brother was not so bright but kind.

The older brother was also a clever businessperson who supported the household with no help from his brother. (The younger brother wanted to help but didn't know how.) Over time, the older brother grew tired of this and told his brother to leave and find his own way to make money. Their mother was so saddened by her oldest son's cruelty, she too left the house that very day.

With no money for a proper home, the mother and son took shelter in an abandoned hut at the foot of a high hill. Early the next morning, the young son took an ax and headed up the hillside to chop wood. By late in the day, he had enough wood to sell in the nearby village, which he did, for a lot of money. The mother and son were relieved to know they had a way to survive.

The following day, the son climbed higher on the hillside to find more fallen limbs for chopping. There, he came upon an impressive surprise—a life-size lion made of stone. He decided this stone guardian of the mountain must be why he'd had such good luck the day before.

The next morning, he lit a candle on either side of the lion, then bowed low before it as he prayed for more good fortune. The lion awoke and asked, "Why are you here?"

The son told the lion his sad story and explained how he wanted to show his gratitude in hope of the lion's continued help. Pleased, the lion said, "Return to me tomorrow, and bring along a big bucket. I will fill it with gold!"

The next day, with bucket in hand, the son bowed low before the lion, who said, "Hold the bucket under my mouth, and I will vomit gold into it. Take care to watch, and when the bucket is almost full, you must tell me. Not a single nugget of gold can fall from the bucket."

The son did exactly as the lion had instructed. After thanking the lion for his generosity, the son set off to show his mother the bucket full of gold. With their fortune, the grateful mother and son settled into a large farmhouse and bought cattle and sheep.

Meanwhile, the older brother showed no interest in the well-being of the family he'd turned away. But when he heard about their newfound fortune, he decided that he and his wife should pay them a visit. The kindhearted, forgiving younger brother gave his unexpected guests a warm welcome and told them how he came to have such wealth. He even urged his brother to seek out the generous lion too.

The next day, carrying the largest bucket he could find, the greedy brother made his way up the hillside. As soon as he found the lion, he lit candles just as his younger brother had directed, then bowed and prayed for good fortune. With that, the stone lion awoke, and the older brother placed a bucket under its mouth. Before he began to vomit gold, the lion warned the brother about keeping a careful eye on the bucket.

The greedy brother's heart jumped as a stream of gold vomit proceeded from the lion's mouth. His selfish spirit put a clamp on his lips, keeping him from telling the lion when the bucket was nearly full. When a piece of gold fell to the ground, the vomiting stopped.

The lion growled. "The largest piece of gold is stuck in my throat. Put your hand into my mouth and pull it out."

Without thinking twice, the brother stuck his hand in the lion's mouth, ready to grab a chunk of gold. Instead, the lion closed his jaws and refused to let go. The horrified brother looked down to see his bucket filled with nothing but rocks and dirt.

By nightfall, the older brother's worried wife went looking for him. A long hillside search brought her to the horrible sight of her husband with his hand stuck in the mouth of a stone lion. She begged for the lion's mercy, but he refused. Finally, the wife walked home and returned with food for her trapped husband. As days, then weeks, then months passed, the weary wife sold more of their belongings until she could no longer afford to bring even a crust of bread to her husband. The couple knew that it was only a matter of time before they would die, and without a coin to their name.

When the lion decided he had taught the greedy son a lesson, his jaws opened wide in laughter. The humbled brother was finally free! He and his wife went straight to his brother's home to beg for help. The younger brother expressed his anger and disappointment before he found it in his heart to show mercy. He gave his brother enough money to buy a simple farmhouse. The kind younger brother went on to live well on his spacious farm, where he took loving care of his mother and found success in all he did.

CHUCK'S SICK SCIENCE

G Is for Gluten Intolerance

 PROFESSOR ANITA PUKE: A person with gluten intolerance may feel nauseous after eating something with gluten in it.

 CHUCK: Can't you just eat around the gluten? I eat around the mushrooms in my mom's cream of kumquat and mushroom soup all the time.

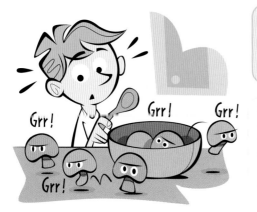

 Gluten is a protein found in wheat and other grains. Wheat is used to make flour. So there's no way to eat around the flour used to make cereal, pasta, and baked goods.

 Baked goods? Hold on . . . you mean cookies. No chocolate chip cookies?! Now I feel nauseous.

 Good news! You can find lots of yummy gluten-free goodies at the grocery store.

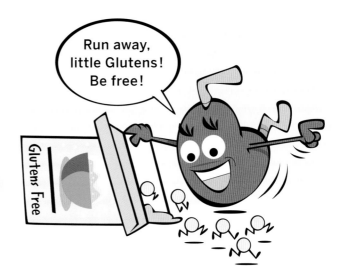

Run away, little Glutens! Be free!

Glutens Free

GLOTTIS

This is the gap between your vocal cords. Air passes through that gap when you breathe. But when you are ready to swallow food or fluid, the vocal cords close like a little curtain to make sure food or fluids do not go into the lungs.

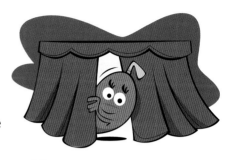

PROFESSOR ANITA PUKE: I'm speechless!

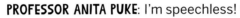

Queezy's Question

How could eating raw cookie dough make me gush?

PROFESSOR ANITA PUKE: Here's how the cookie crumbles: Germs can get into the grain that's used to make flour. But when you make cookie dough with the flour and bake it, the heat of the oven kills the germs. The same is true for raw eggs used to make cookies.

QUEEZY: So unbaked cookies have live germs in them?

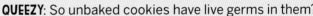

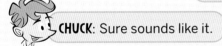
CHUCK: Sure sounds like it.

That makes me want to toss my cookies!

That leaves more cookies for me!

GO TO page 165 to meet the Puking Man—Protector of Flour!

Worst-Ever Family Dinner Ends in War

When the Greek god Kronos became king of the Titans, he received a warning: Someday one of your children will take the throne from you. To protect his job, Kronos swallowed each of his first five children as soon as they were born. When Kronos's wife gave birth to their sixth child, Zeus, she played a trick on Kronos. After hiding newborn Zeus in a cave, she handed her husband a rock wrapped in a blanket. Sure enough, paranoid Kronos swallowed that "baby" too!

When Zeus grew up, he put a special potion in his father's drink that would force him to vomit. Up came Zeus's brothers and sisters, along with that stone infant. With his siblings by his side, Zeus went to battle against Kronos and won. Just as it was foretold, King Kronos lost the throne to one of his own children.

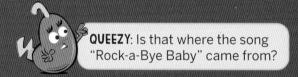

QUEEZY: Is that where the song "Rock-a-Bye Baby" came from?

THE AUTOMATIC GAG

PROFESSOR ANITA PUKE: You know what swallowing is. Gagging is the opposite of swallowing. A gag reflex is a natural response, an action your body does automatically. You don't even need to think about it. If something touches the back of your mouth, the uvula may trigger you to gag or vomit to keep you from choking. That's the way your body protects you from swallowing something that shouldn't be there.

CHUCK: You mean like a fly?

QUEEZY: I know an old lady who swallowed a fly. Hmm. Not sure what happened to her.

MAKE YOUR OWN

Gag Gift

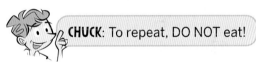

CHUCK: To repeat, DO NOT eat!

Go for a maximum gross factor with this one. It's NOT made to be eaten.

⭐ ***Before you begin:*** Practice food safety (and avoid the vomit). Always start by washing your hands and cleaning the area of the kitchen where you'll be cooking. You'll want an adult to help you. Make sure your assistant has clean hands too!

COLLECT IN A RESEALABLE PLASTIC BAG:

• Cooked oatmeal with a tiny drop of green food coloring added

• Bits of leftovers, chopped into small pieces to look like chewed food

• Piece of chewed gum

• Small plastic fly, rubber band, or toy frog

HERE'S WHAT YOU NEED TO DO:

Seal tight, and mush ingredients together.

Queezy's Tip

"Wrap" your gag gift in a barf bag. See page 26 for instructions on how to make your own.

Great Green Gag Gumbo

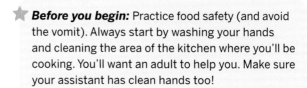

MAKES 1 SERVING FOR A BRAVE PERSON

YOU WILL NEED:

- 1 big scoop mint chocolate chip ice cream
- 1 spoonful of each:
  - Chopped pickles
  - Green olives
  - Green gummy bears
  - Chopped celery
  - Chopped green bell pepper
  - Chopped green onion, lettuce, or kale

Queezy's Tip

If you find someone willing to try this, grab a bucket.

⭐ **Before you begin:** Practice food safety (and avoid the vomit). Always start by washing your hands and cleaning the area of the kitchen where you'll be cooking. You'll want an adult to help you. Make sure your assistant has clean hands too!

HERE'S WHAT YOU NEED TO DO:

Step 1: Put one big scoop of ice cream in a bowl. Let it melt while you prep the rest.

Step 2: Stir in the other ingredients.

Step 3: Top it all off by sprinkling on chopped green onion (or lettuce or kale).

GUESS WHAT? Letter G is about gone. But it gave us enough gross goop to keep us feeling green going into letter H. (Got any ideas who would be grateful to get your gag gift?)

Hey, letter H! Can horses hughie? Do honeybees barf honey? Who has a hunch you can hurl from more than one hole?

Have you heard how you can have the answers? Huh? Head on over to letter H. Hurry!

H

Hello! Happy to have you here! Have you ever wondered **how you hurl**? How about critters who haven't got what it takes to **honk hot air**? Can a frog **holler** in its habitat if its fly holder isn't happy? The answer may turn you inside out!

Hack: unpack the gooey gut sack

Hawk Your Head Off: hurl food with such force, your face goes flying

Heading Out: when squishy food spurts up your throat and out your mouth hole

Heave Up Jonah: open wide like a whale with a salty Jonah ready to bail

Hoist Your Toenails: heave so hard you end up with toes for teeth

Hold the Throne: hold the phone while you fill the throne

Holler: open wide and yell out the yuck

Honk Hot Air: when spicy food calls a fire drill and shoots flames out the face

Hoop: feel what was turning around in the belly roll on out

Hork: when you got a bit too piggy with the pork and spew barbecue

Hughie: spewy in the loo-y

Hurl: feel the food whirl and unfurl out of your face

Queezy's Question

Hey, how do we hurl?

PROFESSOR ANITA PUKE: I love this question, Queezy! Hurling is quite an impressive process. The stomach is equipped with special cells that are on high alert for anything that's unsafe. If those sensor cells detect a problem, they can use a chemical called serotonin to send a message to the nervous system. Once that message is received, it goes straight to the top.

QUEEZY: You mean?

Yes! The brain is where the vomiting center is located. The vomiting center is like the control tower for the whole operation. That's where the command to "hughie" comes from.

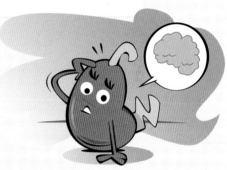

"In three . . . two . . . one . . . we are go for lurch."

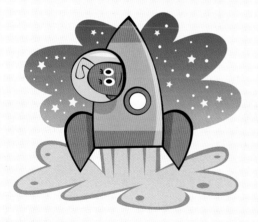

When the command is sent, the stomach muscles shift into crunch mode. The pressure gets more intense. The sphincter muscle that usually does an excellent job keeping food inside your stomach takes a break and relaxes. And the pyloric sphincter muscle that opens to let food leave the stomach and escape into the intestines slams shut. Now there's nowhere for vomit to go but up.

My body does all that without telling me?

That's right. It's protecting you before you even know you need it. But it does give you hints that something's up—or, should I say, is going to come up. Before you vomit, you might get a queasy feeling, and your mouth may fill with extra saliva. Those clues are coming from your brain.

I love how my brain thinks even when I don't.

WONDERING ABOUT the pyloric sphincter muscle?
Flex on over to page 160.

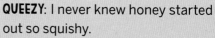

Queezy's Question

I have a sweet question.
Is honey really bee barf?

PROFESSOR ANITA PUKE: No, honey is not bee barf. Honeybees collect nectar from flowers and store it in a special nectar stomach. (It has a separate stomach for food.) When the bee returns to the hive, it regurgitates the nectar mixed with belly fluid (brings it back up into its mouth). Then that mixture is passed from bee to bee to draw out the moisture.

QUEEZY: I never knew honey started out so squishy.

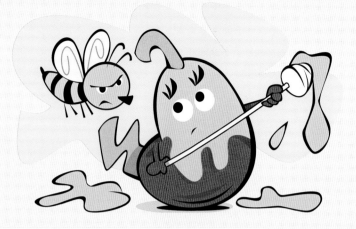

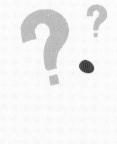

After the "processed" nectar is tucked into the honeycomb, bees fan it with their wings. That makes more moisture evaporate. What's left is thick, sticky honey.

That was a sweet story.

Did You Know?

Would you bee-lieve bee-fore we had medicines made by chemists, honey was used on wounds to help the healing process? And it worked. You'd never try that with insect vomit!

CHUCK'S SICK SCIENCE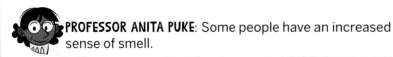

H Is for Hyperosmia

 PROFESSOR ANITA PUKE: Some people have an increased sense of smell.

 CHUCK: Ew. They smell more than other people?

No, they're not smelly. Hyperosmia means you are super-sensitive to smells—both good and bad. The nose of someone with hyperosmia may easily pick up on some odors other noses don't notice.

 Interesting. So, instead of picking your nose, your nose picks smells.

 I never "nose" what you'll say, Chuck! Now, at times, having such a sensitive sniffer could be nice. If you notice the potato salad smells weird, that's a clue it could be spoiled, and you'd know it isn't safe to eat.

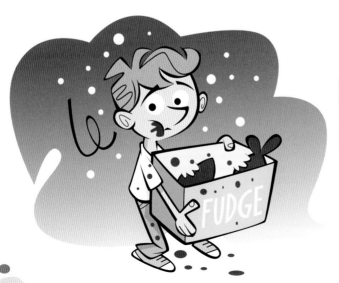

 Almost makes me wish I had hyperosmia. It would have saved me from eating that fish fudge last week.

Now, Chuck, you should have known something smelled fishy about that!

Does hyperosmia have a downside?

Yes. The smells that do bother a person with hyperosmia can make them feel nauseated and trigger a migraine headache. They may vomit too.

Queezy's Question

Are humans the only ones who hork?

PROFESSOR ANITA PUKE: Humans are not the only ones who vomit.

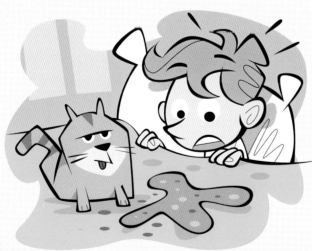

CHUCK: My cat Donut horks on my bed.

QUEEZY: That's crumb-y. "Donut" let him do that.

Many animals, like cats and dogs, can reduce the inventory in their bellies by vomiting. But not all.

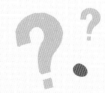

You mean there are animals that have no hurl-ability?

 Indeed. Rodents like mice, rats, and squirrels can't vomit.

 No barf-ability? What about Lickety Split?

 Turtles need water with their food. If not, they may throw up due to tummy trouble.

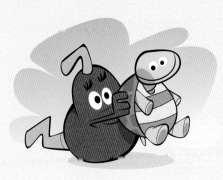

 That's why I feed my turtle in the bathtub!

 Horses can't hurl either. A horse's body is built to keep food from coming back up, even when it gallops.

 What else?

 Because it can't throw up what is in its belly, a frog will throw up its whole stomach.

 Wow!

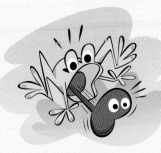

 Then the frog will use its front feet to wipe its stomach off before packing it back inside its body.

 Hey, that's how I clean out my pockets.

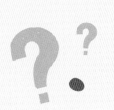

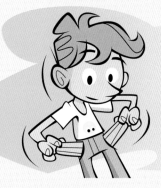

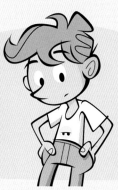

86

CHUCK'S SICK SCIENCE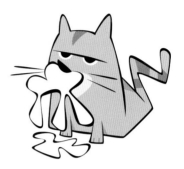

Hypersalivation

The water in your mouth is a fluid called saliva. Ever notice how your mouth fills with extra saliva when you feel nauseous or right before you vomit? Hypersalivation—too much saliva, aka mouthwatering—can be a warning.

SPEAKING OF *mouthwatering . . .*
There's no need to wait for the special day.
Any day—every day—can be a barfday!
Check out page 24 for a recipe.

HOW ABOUT that letter H, huh? Such a hyper letter. Hyperosmia. Hypersalivation.

Impressive letter I is an ideal place for an in-depth investigation of the long and short of the intestines. In addition, it's got the inside scoop on how an icky inner ear can make your insides unhappy. Imagine that!

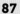

I

Incredible! Letter I includes the inside scoop on the incredible large and small **intestines.** There's incoming ingenious intelligence on *indigestion* and how to *out*smart it. Inspect important instructions on how to make an **interrupting eruption.**

TURN UP THE VOLUME ON YOUR VOMIT VOCABULARY

Ill Will: feel nauseous waiting to see what the stomach will do

Insides Out: when you go out to lunch, and then lunch goes out on you

Insult the Shoes: leak lasagna and splurt spaghetti on your sandals

Interesting Outcome: see what a taco looks like turned inside out

Interior Desecrator: move the stomach's interior to your shirt's exterior

Interrupting Eruption: when the belly bubbles over and breakfast bursts out

Irresistible Purge: when you can't stop unstuffing your stomach

IT TAKES GUTS— SMALL AND LARGE

Small Intestine

Try this: Lay twenty-four sheets of notebook paper out on the floor, short end to short end. That's how long your small intestine will be once you're fully grown—22 feet (6.7 meters) long.

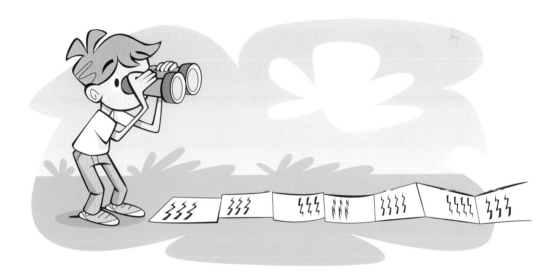

Large Intestine

Try this: Lay seven unsharpened pencils out on the floor end to end. That is the length of the large intestine—5 feet (1.5 meters) long.

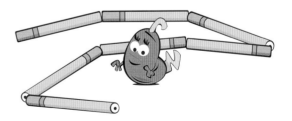

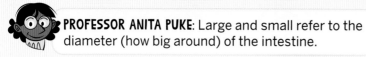

Queezy's Question

Why is the large intestine called large when it's shorter than the small intestine?

PROFESSOR ANITA PUKE: Large and small refer to the diameter (how big around) of the intestine.

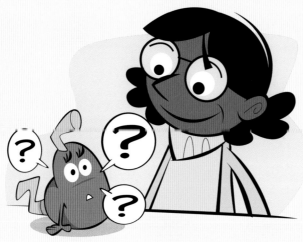

Think of the intestine like two garden hoses. To know which one is small and which one is large, you would measure the opening where the water comes out.

QUEEZY: So the small intestine may be longer, but the large intestine is the biggest intestine "around"!

Get Around to It

Small intestine is 1 inch (25.4 mm) around. Large intestine is 3 inches (76.2 mm) around.

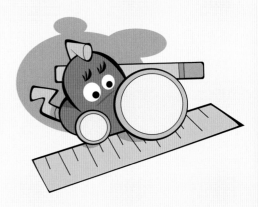

CHUCK'S SICK SCIENCE

I Is for Indigestion

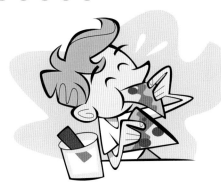

You get home from school and head straight to the fridge. Three pieces of leftover pepperoni pizza have been calling your name since last recess. You're ready to answer that call. On the count of one, two, three, you poke pizza down the shoot. You take a big swig of chocolate moo juice (aka milk) and then grab your bag for soccer practice.

The not-so-funny thing is, when you bend over to put on your shin guards, ew, you feel nauseous. Uh-oh. You've got a case of indigestion, also called dyspepsia. Indigestion is better known as an upset stomach.

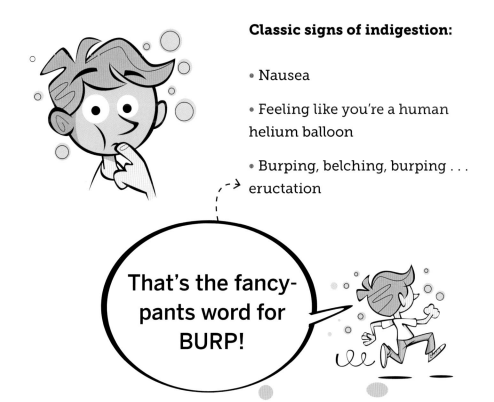

Classic signs of indigestion:

• Nausea

• Feeling like you're a human helium balloon

• Burping, belching, burping . . . eructation

That's the fancy-pants word for BURP!

How to OUTsmart INdigestion

• Eat small meals and go slow.

• Give your belly a bit of time (an hour is best) to digest dinner before you dash.

• Go easy on greasy foods, chocolate, citrus fruits, or any food that makes you feel queasy.

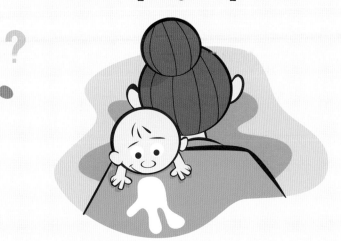

Queezy's Question

Why do infants make so many "interrupting eruptions"?

PROFESSOR ANITA PUKE: Most infants who are only a few months old will spit up after being fed. That's because the muscle between the esophagus . . .

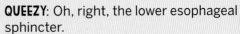**QUEEZY**: Oh, right, the lower esophageal sphincter.

That's correct! That muscle hasn't fully developed yet. Until it can tighten like it should, it's easy for what's in the baby's belly to come back up.

So, it's like toothpaste.

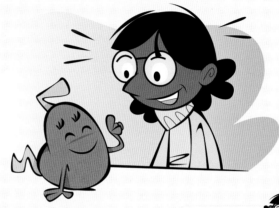

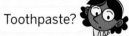Toothpaste?

If you squeeze the tube too tight . . . BLOOP. And that's why I never squeeze a baby.

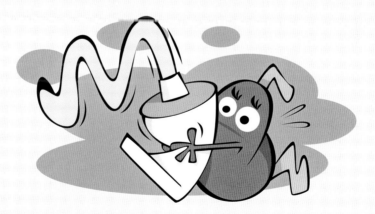

Good news! Most babies stop spitting up after meals by the time they celebrate their first birthday.

95

Emesis Etymology

WHERE DID THAT WORD COME FROM?

Ignivomous

This hot adjective from the Latin of the late 1600s means "vomiting fire." It's a combo of *ignis,* which is Latin for "fire," and *vomere,* "to vomit."

Let's try it in a sentence!

After Chuck poked a pack of flaming pepperoni and dynamite red pepper pizza bites down the shoot, his belly became an ***ignivomous*** volcano.

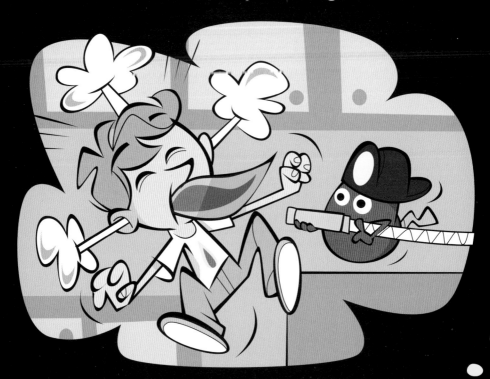

TOUGH ON THE TUMMY

Before You Pump Iron

Iron is a mighty mineral. It powers the body by helping to move oxygen from the lungs to your other precious parts. It also helps muscles store and use oxygen.

If your body is low on iron, you may feel like a limp lump due to a condition called anemia. That means you don't have enough healthy red blood cells to distribute all that energizing.

Not to worry! Iron supplements (taken like a daily vitamin) can give the body the boost it needs. Your doctor can tell you if you need more iron.

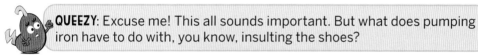

QUEEZY: Excuse me! This all sounds important. But what does pumping iron have to do with, you know, insulting the shoes?

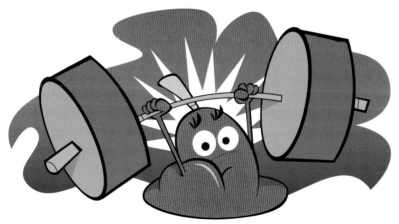

Iron enters the body best on an empty belly. But taking iron can cause cramps and nausea. So eat a small snack before you swallow supplements. (But don't drink milk with the snack! Moo juice makes it harder for the body to soak up iron.)

IBUPROFEN—EASES PAIN, BUT EAT FIRST!

Your parent or doctor may give you a pain reliever like ibuprofen (in the form of tablets, chewables, or liquid) to help you feel more comfortable when you're in pain—like when you have a sore throat or a toothache, or when you get kicked in the elbow at soccer practice.

Ibuprofen can be tough on the tummy. When you take a pain reliever, be sure to eat a snack to avoid getting a painful bellyache (on top of the bruised elbow).

IPECAC SYRUP TO THE RESCUE

Ipecac is sometimes used in an emergency if you accidentally swallow certain kinds of poison. It is specially made to help you throw up to get the poison out of the body as soon as possible.

If you think you may have swallowed poison, it's important to call Poison Control and follow their directions before using ipecac syrup.

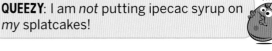

QUEEZY: I am *not* putting ipecac syrup on *my* splatcakes!

FOR A RECIPE to make splatcakes (with *no* ipecac syrup), head over to page 191.

INSTRUCTIONS ON HOW TO "BOWL" (BARF IN A TOILET)

CHUCK: Never barfed? Seems unlikely, but even a puking pro could use a refresher, right?

Let's assume you've made it to the ideal place to puke—the bathroom. Phew! Now what?

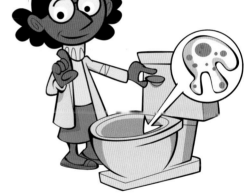

Step 1: Flush the toilet. This will get the inside of the toilet bowl wet. Now you've got a slippy slide for vomit chunks. No sticking!

Step 2: Lift the toilet seat. (You can use toilet paper to cover your hand to avoid touching the seat.)

Step 3a: Bend over the toilet and put your hands on top of the toilet tank (the part that has the flushing device or handle).

or

Step 3b: Kneel in front of the toilet. Try not to lean your arms or hands on the rim of the toilet bowl. (If you feel you really need to, and you have time, do a quick mummy wrap of your hands and arms using toilet paper.)

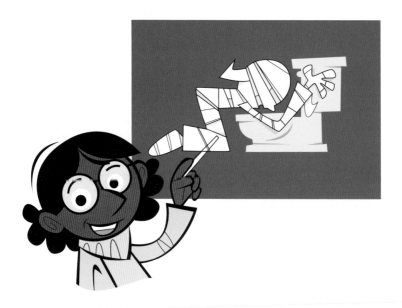

Step 4: Try to get your face right over the toilet bowl to avoid splashing.

Step 5: Let your body do its thing however many times it needs to. Try to relax in between.

Step 6: When you're done, flush the toilet. Close the lid. Wash hands.

If you don't feel well enough to clean up after yourself, that's okay. But be sure to tell someone so they don't get a rude surprise—especially if the "interrupting eruption" makes it outside the toilet.

YOU ERUPTED . . . now what?
Find the next steps toward feeling better
faster on page 145.

Queezy's Question

Did you hear that? What's happening in "ear"?

PROFESSOR ANITA PUKE: The inner ear helps you keep your balance. If your inner ear looks red and feels hot, swollen, and painful, you may feel like your head is spinning. Feeling dizzy could cause you to be nauseous and vomit.

QUEEZY: Sounds *ear*-itating to me.

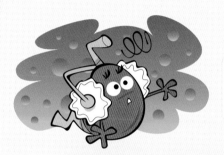

Even if the earache doesn't make you "insult the shoes," it's still a good idea to tell an adult so they can help you with the discomfort.

HEAR! HEAR! For more "ear-formation," visit page 17.

LETTER I was downright irresistible. From the interesting intestines to indigestion zappers to a hot new word (remember what it was?), you increased your VI (vomit intelligence).

Thirsty for more? Just ahead there's a juicy recipe and knock-knock jokes. If it's o-*K*, letter J and letter K will be jumbled together.

Know what? It's time to jump in!

J AND K

No joke! Just for you—a recipe for **Jumble Juice** to jostle the tonsils while you wade into a whale of an epic about **Jonah,** a giant fish, and a jelly-belly-jumbled beach.

Letter K lets you know how to keep away from the germ buffet while you create **Kaleidoscope Cough Cabbage Cones.** Keep up with Hurled History at a **Knossos** palace with a "throne."

TURN UP THE VOLUME ON YOUR VOMIT VOCABULARY

Jelly Belly: jam the belly with too much jelly ("Oops. I made something smelly.")

Jiggly Juice: produce a jiggly pool of cottage cheese and tomato juice

Juggle Jambalaya: stuff yourself with a spicy, ricey mishmash until the belly balks and you spew into the bayou

Jumble Juice: when orange juice pours out your face spout

Jump Shot: when puke bypasses the toilet and detours to the tub

Kaleidoscope Cough: spew a colorful swirl of oranges, blueberries, and green beans

Keep It Moving: bring breakfast back

Kneel Before the Porcelain Throne: bow in front of the barfing bowl

Knock-Knock! Spew's There?: Spew who? Spew better move!

EPICS of EMESIS

Adapted from the Bible's Book of Jonah

Big Fish Barfs Jonah on the Beach

Jonah was given a job by God. He was told to warn a city filled with evil people to change their ways. Jonah didn't want to go. Instead of sailing to the city he was supposed to warn, Jonah jumped in a boat going in the opposite direction.

While on the ship, a terrible storm churned the sea. The crew worried the ship might sink and they'd all drown. Finally, Jonah told the sailors he was running from God. The sailors decided he must be to blame for the wild waves and wind. For the sake of the crew, the sailors tossed Jonah overboard. Right then, the whirling winds stopped, and the water became peaceful. Everyone felt safe again—except for poor Jonah. When he was tossed off the boat, he caught a ride inside a large fish! He spent three days and three nights in a big, wet, stinky belly praying to God to rescue him. God answered Jonah's prayer by ordering the fish to vomit Jonah out onto the beach.

Once again, God told Jonah to go and warn the city of evil people. And that time, he did!

 QUEEZY: I sure hope Jonah took a bath first!

KITCHEN SAFETY TIME

Keep Away from the Germ Buffet

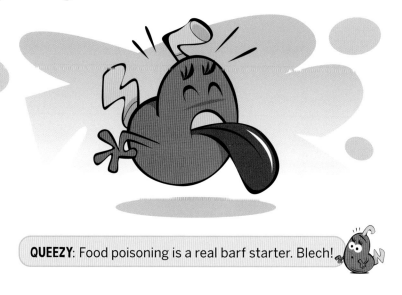

QUEEZY: Food poisoning is a real barf starter. Blech!

To push pause on food poisoning, follow these tips to keep yourself and your family safe:

- **Keep clean.** Wash your hands. Cook with clean spoons, pans, and dishes. Use hot, soapy water to clean kitchen counters before and after making food.

- **Shower and scrub fruits and veggies.** Rinse apples and carrots (and all those crunchy goodies) under running water, especially if you plan to eat them without peeling first.

- **Give food some space.** Even food needs boundaries. Keep raw foods, especially meat, away from cooked food or ready-to-eat foods, like a sandwich or cookies.

- **Only eat baked cookies.** Don't eat raw cookie dough or cake batter.

- **Let cold food chill out.** Refrigerate or freeze foods that can go bad right away.

- **Fling fuzzy food.** If a food you're used to eating looks or smells weird, toss it. It's better to be safe than sick.

WONDER WHY chomping raw cookie dough is a no-no? Find out on page 75.

K IS FOR KINDNESS

If you see someone at school vomit, stay calm. Try not to freak out. Treat the person the way you'd want to be treated if you were the one feeling sick.

- Hand the person a tissue or paper towel and a bottle of water.

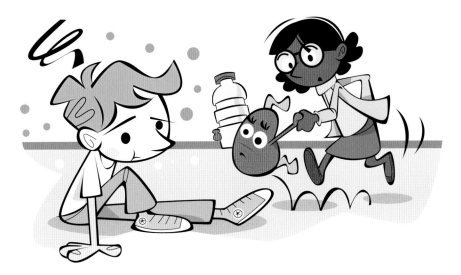

- Find an adult to help, especially if you feel like you're going to get sick too.

- Avoid the urge to laugh at the awkward situation. Instead, be kind. You can both laugh about it—later.

Bonus Barf-eteria Points for Extra Kindness

Want to show a friend with long hair that you care? Offer to hold their hair back to keep it out of their eyes or mouth—and especially away from the toilet. Consider it a rare chance to bond over a belly blowout. Bombing the bathroom is bad enough. No one wants to wear their lunch, much less "wash" their hair in it.

TIME TO LAUGH AT YOUR SHOES

When everybody's feeling better, go ahead and make a joke!

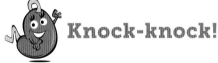

Knock-knock!

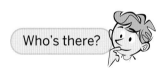

Who's there?

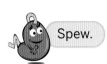

Spew.

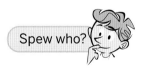

Spew who?

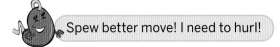

Spew better move! I need to hurl!

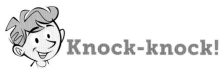

Knock-knock!

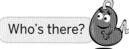

Who's there?

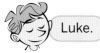

Luke.

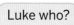

Luke who?

Luke out!
I need to spew again!

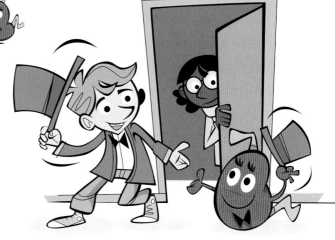

Knock-knock!

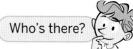

Who's there?

Cashew.

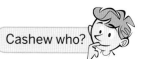

Cashew who?

Cashew see? I spewed on your shoe.

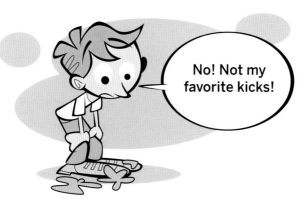

No! Not my favorite kicks!

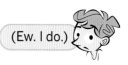

(Ew. I do.)

Kaleidoscope Cough Cabbage Cones

MAKES 4 SERVINGS

YOU WILL NEED:

- 4 empty ice cream cones

FOR CONE FILLING

- 1½ cups shredded purple cabbage
- 1½ cups shredded green cabbage
- 1 heaping cup shredded carrots
- 1 red apple, chopped
- ½ cup dried cranberries
- ½ cup sunflower seeds

Queezy's Tip
If the filling is messy and falls out of the cone, don't worry. Remember, it's a kaleidoscope cough!

FOR DRESSING

- 1½ tablespoons extra virgin olive oil
- 1 tablespoon apple cider vinegar
- 1 tablespoon honey
- ¼ teaspoon salt
- ¼ teaspoon pepper

Before you begin: Practice food safety (and avoid the vomit). Always start by washing your hands and cleaning the area of the kitchen where you'll be cooking. You'll want an adult to help you. Make sure your assistant has clean hands too!

HERE'S WHAT YOU NEED TO DO:

Step 1: Put all the filling ingredients in a big bowl, except for cranberries and sunflower seeds.

Step 2: In a small bowl, mix all the dressing ingredients. Pour the dressing all over the filling and mix it up with a big spoon or tongs. Taste it to see if you want to add a bit more salt or pepper. Cover the bowl with a lid or plastic wrap and put it in the refrigerator for at least an hour.

Step 3: Stir the filling. Use tongs to fill each ice cream cone. Pack it down and pile more on top. Next, sprinkle with cranberries and seeds.

Queezy's Tip
Store leftover slaw (without cones) in the refrigerator for up to five days.

HURLED HISTORY

Welcome to the Palace at Knossos, Home of the Royal Flush

The first place in recorded history where someone could ask: "Okay, who forgot to flush?"

Around 1900 BCE, on the mountainous Greek island of Crete, a palace served as the center of Minoan culture. The walls of the queen's portion of the palace were decorated with murals of dolphins playing in the Mediterranean Sea. But the best part was her "throne room," with the first-known example of a water-flushing toilet.

The wooden toilet seat sat over a drain that could be flushed by pouring water into it from a jug. No, there was no toilet handle like we expect today, but having a toilet that could drain into a closed sanitation system with a sewer (versus hurling into a hole) was a big step up.

 QUEEZY: Big step up? More like a big sit down. And a hurl with no swirl?

Jumble Juice

MAKES ONE 12 OZ. GLASS

 Before you begin: Practice food safety (and avoid the vomit). Always start by washing your hands and cleaning the area of the kitchen where you'll be cooking. You'll want an adult to help you. Make sure your assistant has clean hands too!

YOU WILL NEED:

- 1 cup grape juice (to make 8 frozen juice cubes)
- ⅓ cup orange juice
- ⅓ cup pineapple juice
- ⅓ cup clear soda pop or sparkling water
- Optional: raisins or frozen green peas

Queezy's Tip

Save extra cubes in the freezer for the next time you want Jumble Juice.

HERE'S WHAT YOU NEED TO DO:

Step 1: Drop a raisin or a green pea (or both!) into every slot of an ice cube tray.

Step 2: Pour grape juice into the tray and put it in the freezer.

- When the grape cubes are frozen, it's time to mix the Jumble Juice.

- This drink has four parts—three liquids, plus the grape cubes—so make sure you leave room in the glass for all of them.

Step 3: Drop one or two grape cubes in a tall glass.

Step 4: Pour in the orange juice and pineapple juice. Leave room for the clear soda.

Step 5: Add the soda or sparkling water (slowly!).

JUGGLING LETTER J AND LETTER K—keeping away from the germ buffet, crunching kaleidoscope cones, and journeying in a giant fish. So much knowledge jumping off the page!

Lean in! Legendary letter L lets you learn something "dairy" important about lactose intolerance, plus lumpy burps and loads more.

Let's go!

L

You'll lose your "launch" when you see what's on the list of **lunar litter** that NASA left behind. Learn to say "vomit" in **Latin,** and list **lots of options** for places to **litter the loo** when there's no loo (bathroom) to go to.

Letter L, lead the way!

TURN UP THE VOLUME ON YOUR
VOMIT VOCABULARY

Laugh at Your Shoes: liquefy the laces and soak your funny-looking socks

Leftovers and Out: when the eggs scramble in the stomach and wrestle to be free-range

Liquid Scream: stream ice cream like a bad dream

Litter the Loo: when you set free a deep-dish debris spree ("I thought pizza was my friend.")

Lose Your Lunch: bag up the midday meal and unpack it all over the lunch table

Lumpy Burp: when meatballs retreat and return as *repeat*-balls

Lurch: when your lunch goes out to launch

LUNAR LITTER

The National Aeronautics and Space Administration (NASA) keeps an official catalog of materials from Earth that were left on the moon, like spacecraft vehicles. The list includes a variety of items ranging from a silver medallion to nail clippers to golf balls and even—you guessed it—used barf bags!

Barf Bags Filled per Mission

Apollo 11: 4 bags

Apollo 12: 4 bags

(Apollo 13 didn't land on the moon.)

Apollo 14: 4 bags

Apollo 15: 6 bags

Apollo 16: 1 bag

Apollo 17: 1 bag

Apollo 15 may have used the most barf bags, but to be fair, there's more to the spewy story. The astronauts set records for crewed spaceflight in 1971, including the longest crewed lunar mission (295 hours) and the longest time in lunar orbit (145 hours). It makes sense that more hours spent among the stars meant more chances to spew in space.

CHUCK'S SICK SCIENCE

L Is for Lactose Intolerance

If your body can't fully process the lactose in dairy products like milk, ice cream, and cheese, you may be lactose intolerant. If you are, you can end up with an upset belly, nausea, a bloated feeling, and sometimes even vomiting after eating or drinking dairy.

Lactose intolerance happens if the small intestine doesn't produce enough of an enzyme (lactase) to digest milk sugar (lactose). Without enough lactase to break it down, the milk sugar in the pudding cup you're eating heads right to your colon instead of being processed and absorbed by the body. The colon does not appreciate this because the normal bacteria that live there must interact with all that undigested lactose. That's when the rumbling begins.

If your guts give you grief after eating dairy products, let your grown-up know. Together, you can talk with your doctor about all the good stuff you can eat to stay healthy and avoid post-milk misery.

CHUCK: You can even find stuff like ice cream and chocolate milk with the lactose removed, so you can still make monster milkshakes!

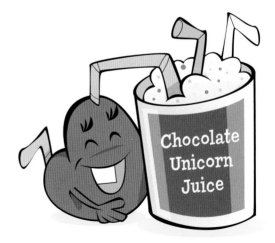

Chocolate Unicorn Juice

LOADS OF OPTIONS FOR AN UNLOADING ZONE

Need to puke but there's no bathroom in sight? Aim for one of these:

- Wastebasket

- Bucket

- Pan or bowl*

- Tall glass

- Flowerpot

- Lunch bag or lunch box

- Backpack

- Plastic shopping bag

- Shoebox

- Sink (only if it's the only option)

Queezy's Tip

Line bowl with a plastic bag, then add some paper towel. That way, you can puke and then pitch it!

Outside? Vomit on grass, not the sidewalk (less spattering and fewer peeved pedestrians!).

Inside? Barf on easier-to-clean tile.

WHAT PALACE provided guests with the first "royal flush"? Roll on over to page 111.

LEARN TO LOSE YOUR LUNCH IN LATIN

Vomo to throw up

Vomito to vomit over and over

Vomitor the person vomiting

Vomitus to belch or spew out

Vomitio the act of vomiting

LETTER L was a real liquid scream! You should feel a lot better now that you have loads of options for where to unload a lumpy burp.

Moving on! Letter M is the messy middle. It mixes the movies, motion sickness, and medieval medicine with a moist hoist. M even mentions how to melt a migraine.

M

Buckle up! Let's take a minute to talk about **motion sickness** on cars, planes, boats, and even your bike. Travel back in time to discover how **medieval** doctors tried to make people feel less miserable. (But it may make you feel sick at the mention of it!) Make time to meet the mighty **medulla oblongata** and the mini-microbe-filled, magnificent **microbiome.**

TURN UP THE VOLUME ON YOUR VOMIT VOCABULARY

Make a Chunky Puddle: cough up mac and cheese and chocolate milk on the crosswalk

Meal-to-Go: when breakfast goes from a takeout bag to a barf bag

Meh Overboard: vomit, but, eh, so what? As in "So I made a chunky puddle. Meh. No big deal."

Messy Middle: when what's inside the middle of you spews down the front of you

Moist Hoist: feel the stomach foist funky tofu

Move Out: pack away pie and have it escape for another try

Mustard Mash: hurl yellowish-green goo after a hot dog or two (or six)

My Lunch Says Hello: bid your burrito goodbye, but then it rebounds

CHUCK'S SICK SCIENCE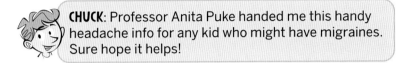

M Is for Migraines

CHUCK: Professor Anita Puke handed me this handy headache info for any kid who might have migraines. Sure hope it helps!

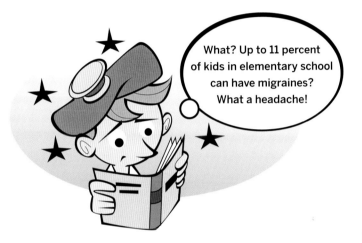

What? Up to 11 percent of kids in elementary school can have migraines? What a headache!

A migraine is a moderate-to-severe headache that can last up to two days, and then come back at least two times a month. These headaches aren't a pain for adults only. Up to 11 percent of kids in elementary school can have them too. Signs of a migraine are not the same for everyone. This list includes more common ones:

• Nausea and vomiting due to pain

• Pounding or throbbing head pain (Kids usually feel pain in the front or on both sides of the head.)

• Pale skin

- Sensitive to sounds and lights

- No appetite

Migraine triggers (the things that get the headache started) are not the same for everyone, but they may include:

- Stress at school

- Too much screen time

- Not getting enough shut-eye

- Skipping meals

- Eating too much processed food with nitrate preservatives like hot dogs, bacon, and lunch meat

- Changes to your routine

- Shift in weather (for example, from warm temperatures to cold and rainy conditions)

- Travel in a car or on a boat

Try melting a migraine headache by . . .

- Using an ice pack on the back of your neck or on the spot where the head hurts.

- Sucking ice chips or sipping water to stay hydrated.

- Staying away from smells or other triggers that might bother you.

- Taking a pain reliever like ibuprofen (with the help of a grown-up).

What if the headache pain heads to your stomach?

Kids are more likely than adults to get what's called an abdominal migraine. Instead of pain in the head, an abdominal migraine causes pain in the stomach. It's usually around the area of the belly button. Researchers are not yet sure what causes this type of migraine, but common triggers include motion sickness, missing sleep, travel, and stress. Taking a pain reliever and resting in a dark, quiet room can help.

HURLED HISTORY

Welcome to Med-"heave"-al Medicine

These people had a weird sense of "humor."

In medieval times, those who practiced medicine followed the teaching of Hippocrates, an ancient Greek philosopher who believed our bodies contained four types of fluid. He called them humors. The humors were blood, phlegm (mucus), black bile, and yellow bile. Nothing funny about those, right? It was believed if you weren't eating right or sleeping enough, your humors could get out of whack, and you could end up with a disease.

To help you get sickly humors out of your body, leeches (a kind of worm) could be placed on the body to suck out the bad blood. Or you might be given a medicine that would make you throw up. Although doctors claimed successes in curing bad coughs, memory loss, and even a diseased liver, sadly, some patients died from these "treatments."

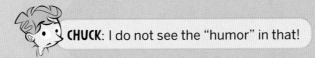 CHUCK: I do not see the "humor" in that!

Queezy's Question

Why do boats cause motion sickness and make passengers blow chunks?

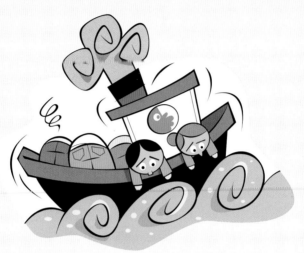

 PROFESSOR ANITA PUKE: *All hands on deck!* It's *a boat* time for a quick quiz!

QUEEZY: I hope I *learned the ropes.* I don't want to feel *dinghy.*

 Remember where we get our sense of balance? Please don't tell me you haven't figured it out *yacht.*

I am *ferry* sure we get our sense of balance from our *oars.* I mean, ears.

 I am *on board* with that answer!

CHUCK: I have a *sinking* feeling, like it *oar* not, you two are going *overboard* with puns.

 Don't *rock the boat,* Chuck!

Professor Puke, it *sailed* past me. How do my ears connect to my gut?

Sorry to *barge* in, but are you saying we can puke out our ears?

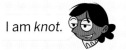
I am *knot.*

Oh, *buoy.* I'm relieved. I was going to wear earmuffs every day.

Imagine you're riding on a boat. Waves move the boat up and down and side to side. The fluid in the inner ear picks up on the motion below the boat, but the eyes can't see what the inner ear is sensing. The brain is confused, and that makes the body stressed. That stress leads to nausea. You may even—

Have a belly blowout on the boat!

Yes. But motion sickness is about more than boats. It can happen in a car, during a bumpy plane flight, on a bike ride, or even when playing virtual games.

I will *drop anchor* right here. I'm never moving again!

Ahoy There! It's Time to Ask Captain Barfbeard!

Q: Do boat captains get seasick?

A: It's said that if you spend enough time at sea, like sailors do, you'll end up in one of two "boats"—people who've *been* seasick or people who *will be* seasick.

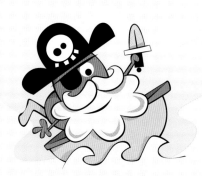

Q: If I get motion sickness easily, can I still become a pilot or a boat captain?

A: Yes, it's still possible to earn your wings, even if you get sick in the air. The same is true for boat captains. Making a moist hoist won't keep you from boarding a plane or a boat.

CHUCK'S SICK SCIENCE

Put the Brakes on Motion Sickness

It can be tough to stop motion sickness once it starts. It's best to keep it from happening in the first place. One of these tips might do the trick:

• Don't eat a big meal before riding in a boat, plane, or car.

• Eat a few dry crackers to settle your stomach.

• Get some fresh air.

• Stay away from strong odors or spicy foods.

• Keep your head as still as possible.

Hey, Chuck, look at me!

No, I can't move my head!

Queezy's Question

Pop the kickstand!
Can you get motion sickness on a bike?

 PROFESSOR ANITA PUKE: Yes, it's possible.

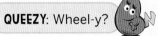 **QUEEZY:** Wheel-y?

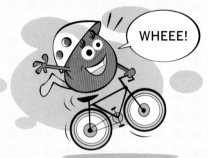 WHEEE!

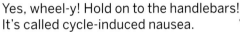 Yes, wheel-y! Hold on to the handlebars! It's called cycle-induced nausea.

Want to avoid cycle-induced nausea? Pop the kickstand and learn how right here:

• **Eat right.** An hour before you plan to bike, eat a small meal that's easy to digest, like eggs and buttered toast, a bowl of oatmeal, white rice, Greek yogurt, or applesauce.

• **Drink right.** Drink plenty of water two hours before you head out. Stay hydrated while you're riding, but don't overdo it.

• **Dress right.** Choose clothes that will protect you from the sun and weather conditions but won't cause you to overheat.

• **Pace right.** Enjoy the ride and don't push yourself too much. Take breaks as needed. Allow yourself to pick up speed and endurance over time.

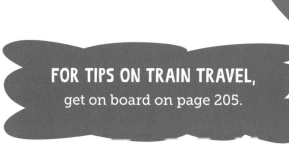

FOR TIPS ON TRAIN TRAVEL,
get on board on page 205.

MOVE OVER, MOTION SICKNESS!

Where are the best seats in the "house"?

For a smoother ride with (hopefully) less motion sickness, sit here:

Boat—Center of the lower deck

Bus—Front seat behind the driver (or upper seating area on a double-decker bus)

Car—Front seat

Plane—Near a wing

Train—First car (or second), facing forward

Motion Picture Outlaw

A rule book called the *Motion Picture Production Code* was enforced from 1930 to 1968. It let moviemakers know what they could and could not show on the big screen. The creators of the code didn't want movie-goers to see anything too gross or upsetting. Filmmakers weren't even allowed to show toilets! Bathrooms and barfing were considered too disgusting and unpleasant for the audience. So that dropped the lid on any scenes with vomit!

Today, vomit is used in so many movies that the Internet Movie Database, better known as IMDb, keeps a list of those films. It's great for people with emetophobia.

HEY, WHAT'S EMETOPHOBIA?
Hurl yourself over to page 56 to find out.

CHUCK'S SICK SCIENCE

Meet the Mighty Medulla Oblongata!

 PROFESSOR ANITA PUKE: I can't wait to talk about your magnificent medulla oblongata!

CHUCK: You're funny. I don't own a fancy sports car. I can't even drive yet!

 The medulla oblongata doesn't sit in a garage. It sits in the lowest part of the brain, at the spot where the brain connects with the spinal cord. It's the manager of some of the most important functions in the body, like your beating heart and breathing lungs.

 That's impressive.

 Not to mention, the medulla oblongata manages your balance, and even—you guessed it—vomiting! That's why the vomiting center is located there.

 Okay, now we're getting somewhere (even if a sports car would get us there faster).

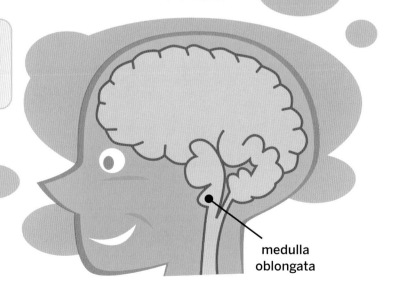

medulla oblongata

When the body is preparing to make a "meal-to-go," the medulla oblongata can trigger you to sweat or make extra saliva or tears. Sweating helps to cool the body. Saliva protects the teeth, and tears protect the eyes.

I'm beginning to see why you think this whole puking process is so cool. Of course, driving a fancy sports car would be much cooler.

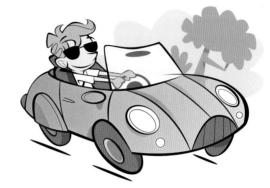

THE MICROBIOME!

It's a good thing a microbe is tiny because the microbiome is made of trillions of them. (Yes, trillions!) Most microbes set up shop in the small and large intestines. And the mix of microbe species is custom to you, thanks to your DNA. Your body met its first microbes as you were being born.

As you grow, you get a greater mix of microbes. Those tiny critters you've collected have been working hard to help your body run smoothly day after day—and most of it is thanks to your own body!

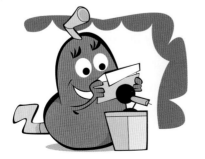

QUEEZY: And the award for Best Supporting Organ goes to . . .

Your Microbiome's To-Do List

☐ Energize the immune system (which protects you from germs that can make you sick)

☐ Break down foods that are hard for the body to digest, like starch and fiber, so the body can put them to good use in preventing health issues and keeping the gut healthy

☐ Provide protection from contaminated water or food

☐ Prevent harmful bacteria from growing too much and competing with your body for the nutrients it needs

How do you like that?

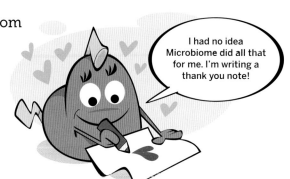

I had no idea Microbiome did all that for me. I'm writing a thank you note!

LETTER M may be messy, but it sure makes you appreciate parts you never knew were in you, like the microbiome and the medulla oblongata.

Need to know more? No problem! Letter N never fails, with nausea, noses, and noni. Never heard of noni? Now you will!

Next up, letter N!

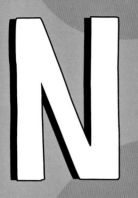

N

Nose way! Why would you *not* want to eat a **noni**? Your nose will tell you. (Noni's nickname gives you a big clue too.) Speaking of nose, true or false: You can **vomit out the nose.** Explore more to sniff out the answer. This may seem like a personal question, but can your **nose** tell you the difference between parmesan cheese and puke?

TURN UP THE VOLUME ON YOUR
VOMIT VOCABULARY

No-Brainer Gut Drainer: before you have a chance to blink, your burrito's in the sink

Nonstop Glop: when the vomit hits repeat

Noot: poke fruit down the shoot and feel a dispute before the gut gives that fruit the boot ("Wah! I liked that kiwi!")

Nose Way: puke out the proboscis (also known as the nose!)

Nowhere to Hide: when the gut puts your gut groceries all out there

Nurffle: overfill, then feel ill till you spill

NONI—VOMIT FRUIT

No Matter What You Call It, This Fruit Stinks

From a tropical evergreen tree grows a lumpy, green, oval-shaped fruit covered in brown dots. It may be small, but it has a hundred regional names, like Indian mulberry, nono, and noni. It's also known by a nickname: vomit fruit. The fruit will not make you hurl, but it will offend the nose!

Not only that, but noni is a fruit that doesn't grow by the rules. Instead of the tree following the typical pattern of producing blossoms first, the fruit grows first, then little white flowers pop out of its brown dots. Once the flowers fall off, the noni begins to ripen, and that's when the stinky business begins. The riper the noni, the paler it looks and the nastier it smells. Some describe the odor as rotting fruit, horseradish, fish, stinky cheese, or vomit (maybe that's all the other smells combined).

In case you're wondering, eating unripe noni is not a good option. True, it's less stinky, but it's too tough to chew and tastes bitter. Ripe noni leaves its aroma in the air, and if you pick noni, its perfume will stay on your clothes and hands.

All that aside, noni fruit does offer health benefits like vitamin C, so some people mix its juice with other fruit juices to get the perks without the P-U! Noni is also appreciated in Polynesian culture for medicinal purposes. It's used to soothe rashes, treat ulcers, and, surprisingly, help with digestion issues. So that doesn't stink.

Did You Know?

My Nose Tastes Funny

Nearly all (almost 80 percent) of what you taste—your favorite fudge ice cream, crunchy tacos, or slurpy noodles—comes from your sense of *smell*. That's why food tastes blah when you have a stuffy nose.

CHUCK: Oh! I get it! So the best time to eat stinky vomit fruit is when your nose is a booger basket.

CHUCK'S SICK SCIENCE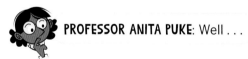

Nausea and Vomiting—What's the Difference?

PROFESSOR ANITA PUKE: Well . . .

CHUCK: Oh! I know this one. Nausea is a gross feeling in my gut. Sometimes it happens right before I upchuck. But not always.

QUEEZY: When you chunder, what's in the gut heads for the exit in the head.

You two surprise me! You're both correct. Nausea is a feeling of sickness, often before you vomit.

Did You Know?

The word *nausea* comes from the Greek word *naus*. *Naus* means "ship sickness."

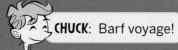 **CHUCK:** Barf voyage!

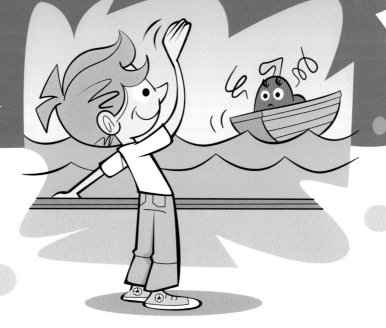

139

Queezy's Question

Is it true you can vomit through the nose?

 PROFESSOR ANITA PUKE: Are you sure you want to know?

 QUEEZY: I'm guessing your question just gave me the answer.

 Yes, it's true. If anybody "nose," it's me! You see, at the end of the soft palate is the uvula.

 Oh, that little punching bag in the throat has a name!

 Yes! That's your uvula. When you breathe with your mouth closed, air goes in the nose, passes over the soft palate and the uvula, and heads to the lungs. The uvula hangs down while that's happening. But when you swallow food or drink, a reflex causes the soft palate to rise, and that closes off the nasal opening at the back of the throat.

 So that's why cereal doesn't go up my nose.

When you laugh or vomit, you exhale, or blow air out. That makes your soft palate and the uvula drop to the breathing position. Vomiting while the uvula and soft palate are in the drop-down position means the liquid coming from the stomach can shoot up your open nasal passages and—

 CHUCK: Spray out your nose!

 Attention, passengers, we apologize for any turbulence. As food begins its descent, please ensure the uvula is in the upright position.

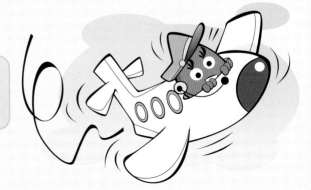

PARM VERSUS PUKE— WOULD YOUR NOSE KNOW?

A Mis-*smelling*, Perhaps? Who "Nose"?

In the early 2000s, Dr. Rachel Herz of Brown University's Department of Psychiatry and Human Behavior wondered if people would react the same way to the same scent if it was placed in identical containers but given different labels.

To find out, she used a chemical combination with butyric acid in it. Butyric acid is a colorless liquid found in dairy products like parmesan cheese—and it's also in human vomit.

To start, Dr. Herz asked participants to sniff from a container labeled "Parmesan Cheese." The reaction was positive. They really liked it.

Next, the participants were asked to smell from a matching container marked "Vomit." The participants didn't even want to take a whiff!

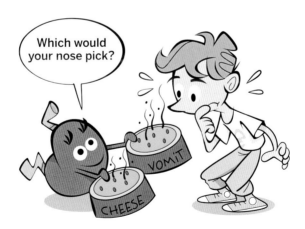

Same smell. Different labels. Very different reactions! Is it a matter of mind over nose? What would happen if you tried this with your friends?

Smells Like Barf, but People Still Buy It

According to the United States Department of Agriculture, Americans eat close to forty pounds of cheese per person in a year. Parmesan is becoming more popular. Cheese sales in the United States reached close to $22 billion in 2022.

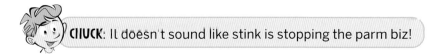

CHUCK: It doesn't sound like stink is stopping the parm biz!

POP UP a pan of stinky, parmy Puke Corn! See page 162.

OH, NO! NOT NOROVIRUS!

Norovirus is a virus that is extremely easy to catch. (A virus of any kind is a type of germ that infects cells and uses them to make copies of itself so it can spread.) Norovirus shows up in the vomit (or poop) of a sick person. So if someone with norovirus uses a bathroom and doesn't wash their hands, anything they touch could have the virus on it.

You can also get norovirus from food that was prepared by someone with norovirus who didn't wash their hands before cooking. And if you happen to be close enough to someone with the virus who is vomiting, you can even potentially breathe in the virus.

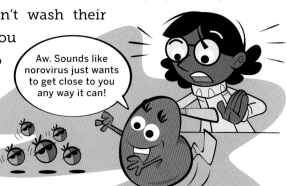

Aw. Sounds like norovirus just wants to get close to you any way it can!

Also, good to know—you can spread norovirus before you even show signs of being sick. The virus spreads easily in places where lots of people get together, like school, a sporting event, a concert, or a cruise ship.

Signs of Norovirus

Norovirus is caused by a germ that can spread from person to person very quickly.

Signs of norovirus include:

- Nausea

- Vomiting

- Diarrhea

- May also cause fever, chills, and headache

If you have a lot of vomiting and diarrhea, it can make you dehydrated and dizzy too.

Under the Weather? Get Over It Faster

There's no vaccine to protect you from norovirus. That means the best way to avoid getting sick is by eating nutritious foods, getting rest, and washing your hands well. Most people with norovirus get better within two to three days and don't need to go to the doctor.

FEEL BETTER FASTER BY:

- Getting lots of rest and drinking plenty of fluids.

- Eating only a little bit at a time and sticking to "blah" foods once you've stopped vomiting. (See the No-More-Nausea Menu on the next page for ideas.) You can eat more as you feel up to it. Don't push yourself. You don't want to prompt more puking.

Did You Know?
Stop Norovirus from Spreading!

Wash your hands well with soap and water, and make sure your family washes their hands too, especially the people taking care of you.

Stay home from school and any public places until the norovirus symptoms (like vomiting) have stopped for at least twenty-four hours.

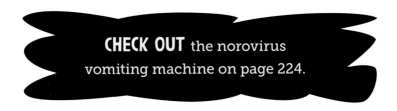

CHECK OUT the norovirus vomiting machine on page 224.

TRY THE NO-MORE-NAUSEA MENU

To reduce that dizzy, nauseous feeling, get some rest, drink lots of fluids, and choose "blah" foods that won't freak out your stomach.

These gentle foods are good choices:

- Vegetable or chicken broth with saltine crackers

- Dry toast (no butter)

- Oatmeal

- Pudding or custard

If you still feel nauseated, sip small amounts of clear, sweetened liquids, such as sports drinks or ginger ale. Skip solid foods. Lie down when you feel dizzy or nauseous, and don't get up until those feelings go away.

When you feel ready to stand, take your time. Go slow to keep from making dizziness worse.

READY TO REHYDRATE? See page 48 for more fluid-refilling options after you're sick.

Did You Know?

After you wash your hands and dry off with a paper towel, you can avoid touching germ-covered bathroom door handles. It's easy. Open the door with a paper towel in your hand.

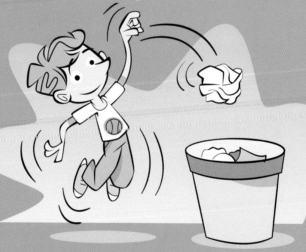

Toss that "germ guard" in the trash nearest the door as you walk out. Score!

NEW WORD ALERT!

Introducing ... **Nauselated**

Really happy + totally frazzled + ready to hurl = Nauselated

This new word was invented by the author of this book.

 QUEEZY: The only time I feel nauselated is when I'm awake. (Or dreaming. Or if there's gravity.)

OKAY, LETTER N! No more talk of nausea, noni, and norovirus (for now!). Don't get too nauselated, but the next letter is covered in oysters!

Only letter O could open with its nose in a book. (You'll see!) Then on to orange vomit and odd body words, oh my! (And yes, oysters.)

On we go to letter "Oh"!

O

What's got an odd fascination with the nose (and other body parts!) and an explanation for **orange vomit,** but won't clam up about **oysters**? You get one guess! Too bad **olfactory senses** can't help when it comes to picking a safe oyster.

TURN UP THE VOLUME ON YOUR VOMIT VOCABULARY

Oodles o' Noodles: what happens when spaghetti is ready to retreat, as in "Oops. My pasta popped out. I made oodles o' noodles!"

Open Wide for What's Inside: when the fried squid you tried slides back outside

Out Spout: churn out vomit from the snout

Over and Out: gross out when leftover brussels sprouts abruptly leak out

Overweight Burp: belch with a hefty surprise ending

CHUCK'S SICK SCIENCE

O Is for Olfactory

 CHUCK: Queezy thinks she *nose* about this one.

 QUEEZY: The olfactory is an old factory where smells are made.

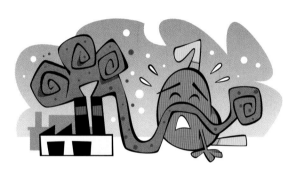

PROFESSOR ANITA PUKE: Hmm. Nice try. I won't say your answer stinks, but it's not on the nose. *Olfactory* refers to the sensory system the body uses for smelling. The sense of smell can sometimes trigger nausea for people with sensitive noses.

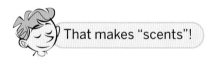 That makes "scents"!

Some people even suffer from osmophobia. It's not that they fear scents, but they do have an extreme disgust for certain smells and odors. The person may smell something like smoke or a cleaning product, and that will trigger a migraine headache. Once the headache is underway, nausea and vomiting can follow.

 Well, that does stink!

You're right on the nose about that one!

 Queezy, you're ready for the U.S. *Nasal* Academy!

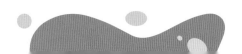

HEY! DON'T CLAM UP.
LET'S TALK ABOUT . . . OYSTERS

Oysters are mollusks that live in salt water, like the ocean. People who like seafood—lobster, shrimp, or clams—may also enjoy eating oysters. Lobster is typically boiled before it's served, but some people eat other shellfish, like oysters, raw.

Here's the tricky part: Eating raw or undercooked oysters can be risky. You could be infected with bacteria that makes its home where oysters do. When oysters feed, they suck in water, keep whatever is edible, and let the water back out, like a filter. When oysters do this, bacteria get pulled in and trapped. That means bacteria can build up inside the oyster. Once bacteria enter a raw-oyster eater's body, they might feel like they swallowed a hurricane because dinner will come up in a tidal wave.

Knowing if an oyster in its shell is safe to eat is tricky because an oyster containing harmful bacteria looks, smells, and tastes just like one that's okay. The only way to make sure any bacteria are killed is to cook oysters properly. Boil them in water until the shells pop open, and then boil for up to five minutes longer. If an oyster's shell stays shut after boiling, keep your mouth shut. In other words, don't eat it! Oysters that have been shucked (removed from the shell) must be boiled, fried, or broiled for at least three minutes to reduce your risk of infection. You can still eat oysters. Just be careful!

I'll have a grilled cheese, please.

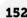

OH! ORANGE VOMIT

The first few times you vomit can bring up food that hasn't made it all the way through the digestion process. That's why you may notice an offensive orangey color.

ODD BODY WORDS

Borborygmic [bor-boh-RIG-mick]: stomach growling. The belly makes that rumbly, grumbling sound all the time. It's easier to hear when your stomach is on "E."

Duodenum [doo-uh-DEE-num]: start of the small intestine, situated between the stomach and jejunum

Hallux [HAL-lucks]: the top toe, the big piggy. That's right—it's the big toe, which helps you keep your balance, even when you're seasick.

Jejunum [jeh-JOO-num]: the second part of the small intestine

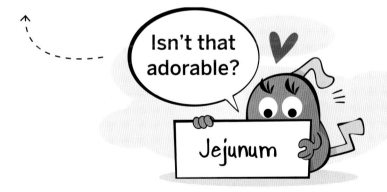

Isn't that adorable?

Jejunum

Philtrum [FILL-trum]: the little groove between the bottom of the nose and the lips. From the Greek word for "love charm," the philtrum has a front-row seat to your puking!

Uvula [YOOV-yoo-luh]: means "little grape" in Latin, and humans are the only ones who have one. If you open wide in front of a mirror, you can see your uvula dangling there at the back.

HANG AROUND page 112 and you'll see there's so much more to know about the little uvula.

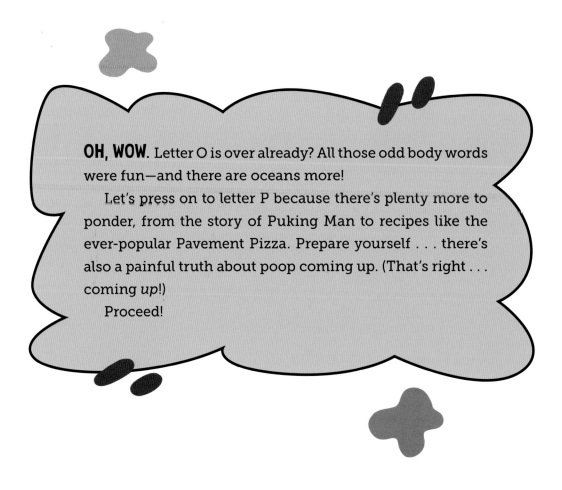

OH, WOW. Letter O is over already? All those odd body words were fun—and there are oceans more!

Let's press on to letter P because there's plenty more to ponder, from the story of Puking Man to recipes like the ever-popular Pavement Pizza. Prepare yourself . . . there's also a painful truth about poop coming up. (That's right . . . coming *up*!)

Proceed!

P

Pass the **Pavement Pizza** and prepare yourself for letter P! This portion is positively puke-packed! So pass the **Puke Punch** and find out who first hurled the word **puke** into the world. Peruse Professor Anita Puke's favorite **parfait** recipe (plus plenty of others!), and pause for the pukey particulars about **projectile vomit.** And our patient professor will get to the bottom of Queezy's question: Can you throw up **poop**?

TURN UP THE VOLUME ON YOUR VOMIT VOCABULARY

Paint the Walls: when stomach matter climbs up the ladder to splatter and scatter

Park at the Porcelain Pool: when puke uses the tongue for a diving board

Pavement Pizza: deliver pepperoni and extra cheese to the sidewalk

Perk: when the belly becomes alert because it's about to spurt

Plornk: plunk the potbelly's bloat overboard

Plummet: catapult a plum (or six) from the tum

Pour the Punch: purge purple party punch in the bowl

Puddle Pudding: when curdled custard spurts like mustard

Puke: revisit your rigatoni, ramen, rice, or macaroni

Queezy's Question

Why do our bodies make puddle pudding in the first place?

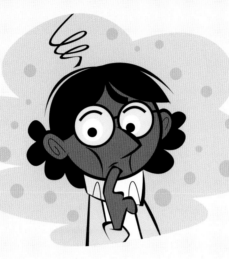

PROFESSOR ANITA PUKE: It doesn't feel great when it's happening, but vomiting is one of the ways your amazing body protects you from threats like viruses, germs, bacteria, or toxic chemicals. Once the body sends a message to the brain about a dangerous invader, a chain reaction removes the unwelcome substance from the body.

QUEEZY: Whoa. It's like I have a built-in bodyguard that saves me a visit to the doctor.

EVER WONDER what goes on in your body when you "pour the punch"? Check out page 236 for insider information.

Professor Puke's Pavement Pizza

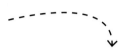

MAKES 6 SERVINGS

YOU WILL NEED:

- 6 mini-pizza-size crusts (English muffins split in half, naan, or biscuits)
- Pizza toppings—pick your favorites
- 1 jar white pizza sauce or queso sauce
- 1 cup shredded mozzarella cheese
- ¼ cup pesto, pickle relish, or chopped pickles

⭐ *Before you begin:* Practice food safety (and avoid the vomit). Always start by washing your hands and cleaning the area of the kitchen where you'll be cooking. You'll want an adult to help you. Make sure your assistant has clean hands too!

HERE'S WHAT YOU NEED TO DO:

Step 1: Preheat the oven to 400 degrees. While the oven gets hot, put the pizza crusts on a baking sheet. Tip: If you are using English muffins, put them in the oven for two to three minutes to toast a bit before adding the toppings.

Step 2: On a cutting board, chop the pizza toppings into small chunks or pieces. Watch your fingers!

Step 3: Dump all the chopped toppings, the white pizza sauce, and the cheese into a big bowl. Mix.

Step 4: Spoon the topping mixture on a pizza crust, then use the back of the big spoon to spread it to the edge of crust.

Queezy's Tip

Store any leftover pavement pizza in a container with a tight lid. Pop it in the freezer. Reheat it in the microwave for lunch or snacks.

Step 5: Bake for 8 to 10 minutes or until the topping mixture bubbles.

Step 6: Remove the pizzas from the oven. Let them cool for 5 minutes.

Step 7: Drizzle a little pesto on top for glistening green pavement pizza.

HURLED HISTORY

No Public Puking in Persia

In 430 BCE, the Greek historian Herodotus compared the culture of his home country with that of Persia (now the country of Iran). Wealthy Greeks were comfortable with guests vomiting at their fancy banquets. Persians, on the other hand, were forbidden from "losing their lunch" in public. Herodotus doesn't mention a fine for breaking the rule, but perhaps Persians thought the embarrassment of accidental public puking was punishment enough.

PYLORIC SPHINCTER

The pyloric sphincter is a ring of smooth muscle at the lower end of the stomach. It connects the belly with the small intestine and controls the travels of partly digested food and stomach juices. When it gets its cue from the vomiting center in the brain, that muscle will tighten to let what's in the gut come right on up.

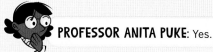

Queezy's Question

Let's get to the bottom of this!
Can I throw up poop?

 PROFESSOR ANITA PUKE: Yes.

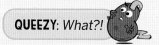 **QUEEZY:** *What?!*

This is known as feculent vomiting. It is rare. But throwing up feces is just like typical vomiting.

 But with the bonus of poop breath!

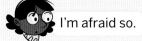 I'm afraid so.

 How could that happen?

 A person might have feculent vomiting if there is a blockage in their intestine. The blockage could be caused by scar tissue, swelling, a hardened mass of poop, or a twisted intestine.

 Wow. How awful! That stinks.

Puke Punch

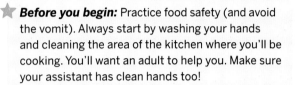

MAKES 6 SERVINGS

YOU WILL NEED:

- 6 cups red fruit punch
- ½ cup cottage cheese
- 2 chopped bananas
- ½ cup blueberries or globs of grape jelly

Before you begin: Practice food safety (and avoid the vomit). Always start by washing your hands and cleaning the area of the kitchen where you'll be cooking. You'll want an adult to help you. Make sure your assistant has clean hands too!

HERE'S WHAT YOU NEED TO DO:

Step 1: Pour ingredients into a clean plastic bucket and stir.

Step 2: Cover top with plastic wrap.

Step 3: Chill in refrigerator.

Step 4: Stir again before serving.

Step 5: Scoop into cups.

Queezy's Tip

Prevent food poisoning: Put any leftover Puke Punch back into the refrigerator. You don't want the guests to make actual puke punch after they leave the party.

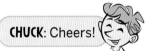

CHUCK: Cheers!

Puke Corn

MAKES 4 SERVINGS

YOU WILL NEED:

- 2 tablespoons vegetable oil (do not use olive oil)
- 1/3 cup popcorn kernels
- 2 tablespoons butter
- Grated parmesan cheese

Before you begin: Practice food safety (and avoid the vomit). Always start by washing your hands and cleaning the area of the kitchen where you'll be cooking. You'll want an adult to help you. Make sure your assistant has clean hands too!

HERE'S WHAT YOU NEED TO DO:

Step 1: Put a large pot on the stove. (You'll need the lid too.) Add the oil and ONE popcorn kernel. (That's your official "test kernel.")

Step 2: Put the lid on the pot and turn the heat to medium-high. Wait for the test kernel to *pop!*

Step 3: Pour in the remaining kernels. Careful! The oil is hot! Put the lid on and swirl the pan to cover the kernels in oil.

Step 4: Listen for popping to start. Give the pot one more swirl.

Step 5: Once kernels *PoP-pOp-Pop-POP!*, crack the lid a bit to let steam out. (Don't open too much, or the oil won't stay hot enough to finish popping the kernels.)

Step 6: When you hear about one pop per second, turn off the heat. (Wait a few more seconds for any late poppers.) Take the lid off and pour the popcorn into a big bowl.

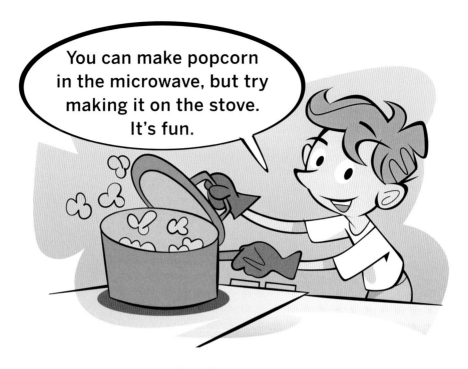

You can make popcorn in the microwave, but try making it on the stove. It's fun.

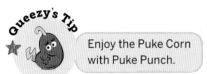
Step 7: Let the pan cool two minutes, then plop in butter. No need to turn on the stove. The warm pan will melt butter.

Step 8: Drizzle butter over the popcorn.

Step 9: Now, for secret Puke Corn ingredient! Sprinkle the popcorn with stinky parmesan cheese.

Step 10: Scoop Puke Corn into smaller bowls to share.

Start the Day with a Puke Parfait

Great for Barf-fest or Brunch!

MAKES 2 SERVINGS

YOU WILL NEED:

- 1 cup plain yogurt
- 2 tall glasses
- 1 cup chopped fresh or dried fruit
- 2 tablespoons honey
- ¼ cup whole grain breakfast cereal

HERE'S WHAT YOU NEED TO DO:

Step 1: Put ¼ cup of yogurt into each glass.

Step 2: Top with ¼ cup fruit.

Step 3: Pour in 1 tablespoon honey.

Step 4: Top with ¼ cup yogurt.

Step 5: Sprinkle with cereal.

Queezy's Tip

Keep in the refrigerator until you are ready to dig in.

Willkommen (Welcome)
the Puking Man of Germany

In the 1500s, mechanically milled white flour was fed into a long, tube-shaped bag. The bag was shaken to set the fine flour free to fall into a wooden box. The unwanted outer shell of the grain (called bran) came out the end of the long bag through a wooden chute and into a trough below.

Here's where it gets interesting. If you gave that wooden chute a second look, you might wonder if you're seeing things. Is that a man's face? Meet Kleiekotzer, the Bran Puking Man. See, at the base of that chute was the image of a wooden masked worker who captures ground-up bran and "pukes" it out of his wide mouth. Using Kleiekotzer to puke out the bran not only purified that year's wheat harvest, but it was also believed to shoo away evil spirits that may infect the bran and grains. These demons, it was said, could cause death or make people who ate the foul flour act wild and see things that weren't there.

Today, we know bran and grains, such as rye, can be infected with fungus (not evil spirits). Eating infected rye flour can result in a medical condition that can cause—you guessed it—hallucinations, which means seeing things that aren't there!

Queezy's Question

Why does vomit fly out of your face?

PROFESSOR ANITA PUKE: It takes a coordinated effort for the body to get what's in the gut back out of the mouth to make pavement pizza. Sometimes, if a person has certain medical conditions, overeats, or has an infection, projectile vomit will come up with a lot more force and without warning. It can send vomit several feet across the room.

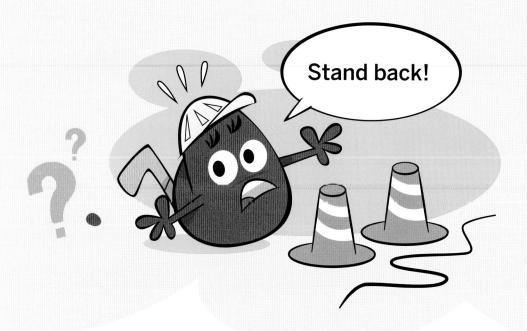

Stand back!

Emesis Etymology

WHERE DID THAT WORD COME FROM?

Whence did the word puke cometh?

PROFESSOR ANITA PUKE: The word *puking* was likely an English version of the German word *spucken,* meaning "to spit." In 1598, the English playwright William Shakespeare used the term *puke-stocking* in his play *Henry IV.* The actual word *puking* showed up in Shakespeare's comedy *As You Like It.*

CHUCK: Can we go back to the "puke-stocking" part?

When Mr. Shakespeare wrote his play, puke was a fancy fabric used to make stockings. Stockings were like heavy tights worn by both men and women to keep warm. This use of the word *puke* came from the Dutch word *puuc,* meaning "the best grade of cloth."

From William Shakespeare's play *As You Like It*

All the world's a stage,
And all the men and women merely players;
They have their exits and their entrances,
And one man in his time plays many parts,
His acts being seven ages. At first the infant,

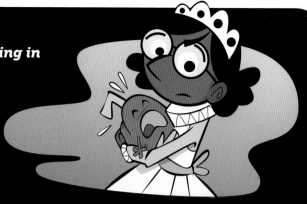

*Mewling [crying] and **puking in the nurse's arms.***
Then the whining schoolboy, with his satchel
And shining morning face, creeping like snail
Unwillingly to school.

Who Knew Vomit Was That Old?

According to the *Oxford English Dictionary*, the word *vomit* appeared in English literature as early as 1529, when Henry VIII was king of England. He and his court enjoyed lavish banquets with as many as twenty choices of fresh meats such as swan, wild boar, eel, porpoise, lamb, peacock, badger, pig, partridge, ox, pigeon, beaver, blackbird, duck, rabbit, quail, salmon, chicken, sparrow, pheasant, and deer seasoned with spices and oils from around the world. But wait, there's more! Guests were stuffed with asparagus covered in a rich sauce, strawberries, breads, puddings, meat pies, custard, plum tarts, jelly, candied fruit, fritters, gingerbread, sugared almonds, and spiced fruitcake. (And everyone ate with their hands!)

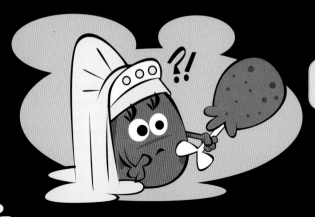

QUEEZY: Um. No wonder they needed the word *vomit*.

Queezy's Question

Can my pet make me puke?

PROFESSOR ANITA PUKE: Pets don't want to make us sick, but they can. Cats, dogs, and reptiles like a pet snake, tortoise, chameleon, or gecko can pass along germs that live in their intestines. The germs can lead to a salmonella infection, causing stomach cramps, nausea, and vomiting.

QUEEZY: Hmm. I should stop licking Lickety Split. He's my pet turtle.

Keep from getting sick by washing your hands well after you pick up your dog's poop, scoop your cat's litter box, or clean your reptile's tank.

Uh-oh. I've only been washing my turtle's hands.

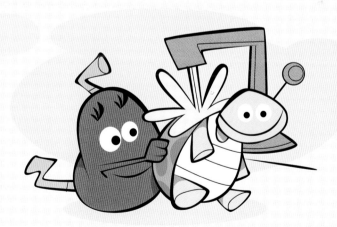

CHUCK'S SICK SCIENCE

Power of Peristalsis

Let's say you eat a frosted doughnut with sprinkles and then do a head-stand. (You know, like you always do!) Will the body still be able to move

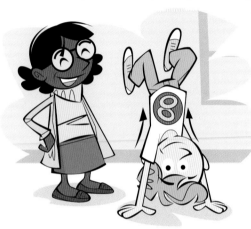

the sweet treat through the digestive system, even against the mighty forces of gravity? Yes! Peristalsis doesn't depend on gravity.

Like an amazing conveyor belt, the stomach contracts (squeezes) to create waves that keep that doughnut rolling along.

CHUCK: It's all about the mighty muscles!

LETTER P proved it has the power to deliver on its promise! Poppin' Puke Corn, a puking man, and projectile puke—it was positively puke-tacular!

You're already in the third quarter of the alphabet! The quirky quest to the quintessential letter Q is only a page away. And you're quite qualified to take a not-so-quick look!

Q

Welcome to high-quality letter Q! Ready to quiz your **spew IQ**? You may get a sinking feeling when you read about **Queen Mary**'s sick ship. But don't quit! Continue your quest to learn how many **quarts** of food your stomach can hold.

TURN UP THE VOLUME ON YOUR VOMIT VOCABULARY

Quack: when your snack ducks out

Quaggy Gaggy: time for the mushy to go flushy

Quake and Shake: shiver and quiver while barfing onions and liver

Quark: quack in the park after dark (see also **Quack**)

Queasy Sneezy: when your stomach feels full of meatball yo-yos and you "sneeze" all over the pillows

Quick Getaway: when dessert decides to dash

Quick Sick: when you had a quack-tree shirt a split second before (see also **Quack**)

HURLED HISTORY

Queen Mary 2—Shipshape or Sick Ship?

The Saga of a Not-So-Bon Voyage

The cruise ship *Queen Mary 2* took 2,613 passengers on a holiday voyage from December 22, 2012, to January 3, 2013. Unfortunately, a "Mr. Norovirus" came aboard as well. In total, 204 of the passengers reported being ill with vomiting and diarrhea, and 16 crew members got sick too.

SAIL OVER to page 126 for seasickness.

GET THE SCOOP on steps you can take to prevent norovirus on page 144.

Queezy's Question

Kids versus adults— who makes more technicolor yawns?

PROFESSOR ANITA PUKE: Kids are exposed to a lot of viruses whenever they hang out together, play sports, and go to school. It takes time for a child's body to build up the same kind of immunity (protection from harmful diseases) that adults have. Because of this, children will vomit more often than adults.

QUEEZY: Woo-hoo! We win! Cookies for all the kids!

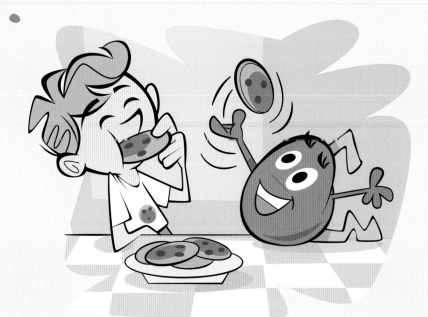

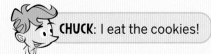

CHUCK: I eat the cookies!

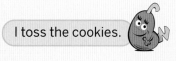

I toss the cookies.

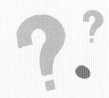

Did You Know?
Hold It!

Four Quarts
That's how much food and liquid most stomachs can hold (or unload!).
FYI: 4 quarts = 1 gallon/3.8 liters

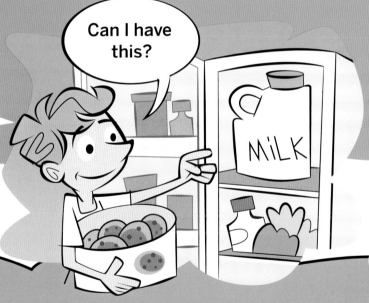

Can I have this?

MILK

LETTER Q was quite quick! How did you do with your spew IQ?

Running on E? Think of letter R like a rest stop. You can learn how to really relax, then reel in the recipe for Ralphabet Goop. (It's not revolting!) Ready?

R

Ready for relief? Read the best ways to **relax** your nervous belly and **rehydrate** after you **ralph on a roller coaster.** And for a real treat, make room for a Ralph-worthy Recipe— **Ralphabet Goop.**

TURN UP THE VOLUME ON YOUR VOMIT VOCABULARY

Rainbow Retch: top off the porcelain pot at the end of the rainbow

Ralph: Ruth

Ralph on a Roller Coaster: fill up, then feel down when the stomach does a corkscrew

Recall: bring a meal back after the buffet

Restroom Karaoke: sing into the potty after too much pizza at a party

Return for a Refund: purchase a meal, eat it, and have it come back on you

Reverse Gears: when wheels in the gut go round and round the wrong way

Rup: have a belly ready to burst, as in "Stand back! He's ready to rup!"

Ruth: Ralph (see also **Ralph on a Roller Coaster**)

Queezy's Question

Ugh! Why does stress make me nauseous?

PROFESSOR ANITA PUKE: First, you should know you're not alone. Lots of people have a physical reaction to feeling anxious.

Here are some things that might help to calm you down:

Be mindful. Breathe. When your mind and heart are racing and your stomach is doing flip-flops, it's easy to feel like everything is out of control. Instead of thinking about what may or may not happen in the future, pay attention to where you are in that moment. If you're in a chair, for example, pay attention to how it feels to press your spine against the back of the chair. Let both feet rest on the floor. Rest your hands in your lap. All you need to do is "be" in that moment.

Be connected. Tell a friend or an adult you trust how you're feeling. It can help you to feel less alone with your anxious thoughts. Your friend may not be able to help you figure out why you feel so stressed, but they can give you a hug (if you want one) and even make you laugh. You can do the same for your friend when they feel frazzled and need to share.

Be thankful. Focusing on the good things in your life can help you break the habit of paying more attention to what stresses you. For example, think about riding bikes with your friends or snuggling your new puppy, watching your favorite funny movie, or even staring up at the stars before you go to bed.

Be rested. Kids ages six to twelve need nine to twelve hours of sleep every night. Being well rested gives you the mental energy to deal with anxious thoughts that cause you to feel nauseous.

SOMETIMES THE EASIEST WAY

to relieve stress and that dizzy, nauseous feeling is to breathe. Page 49 gives you a simple deep-breathing exercise. Try it.

Queezy's Question

Regurgitate. Retch. "Reverse gears." They're all the same, right?

PROFESSOR ANITA PUKE: Same? No. Related? Yes. Regurgitation is a bit like eating in reverse. Swallowed food comes back up the esophagus and into the mouth without warning.

QUEEZY: Oh! So it's like, "We're back! Anyone want a second helping?"

Yes, that's it! Retching is also called dry heaving. It feels like you're going to vomit. You may feel nauseous and retch (make the sounds or movement of throwing up), but nothing comes out. Sometimes a dry heave can lead to real vomiting, but not always.

Ew. So dry heaving is a "retch rehearsal" for vomiting.

 Exactly. It's puke practice! Now, when you "reverse gears" or vomit, that's like a full-scale "evacuation."

Sure, I get it. "Everybody out of the pool!"

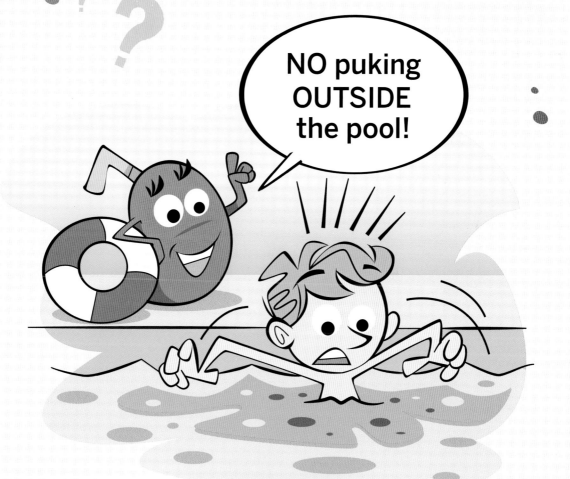

Ralphabet Goop

MAKES 2 SERVINGS

YOU WILL NEED:

- 1 can cream of mushroom soup
- 1 can alphabet noodle soup
- 1 cup frozen or canned mixed vegetables, with water drained
- 1 shake of salt and pepper
- Food coloring—green and yellow are good choices

Bonus: Add one mystery ingredient no one expects to find in soup, like sliced canned pears, olives, or raisins!

⭐ **Before you begin:** Practice food safety (and avoid the vomit). Always start by washing your hands and cleaning the area of the kitchen where you'll be cooking. You'll want an adult to help you. Make sure your assistant has clean hands too!

HERE'S WHAT YOU NEED TO DO:

Step 1: Put both cans of soup, the vegetables, and half a soup can of water in a medium-size saucepan. Add a shake of salt and pepper. Stir.

Step 2: Cook soup over low heat until hot.

Step 3: Add one drop of green food coloring and one drop of yellow. Stir.

Step 4: Turn off the heat. Scoop the goop into bowls.

Queezy's Tip

Just before serving, sprinkle the mystery ingredient over the goop and stir it in.

To show your thanks, make/let your assistant take the first taste!

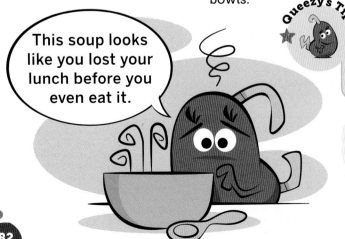

This soup looks like you lost your lunch before you even eat it.

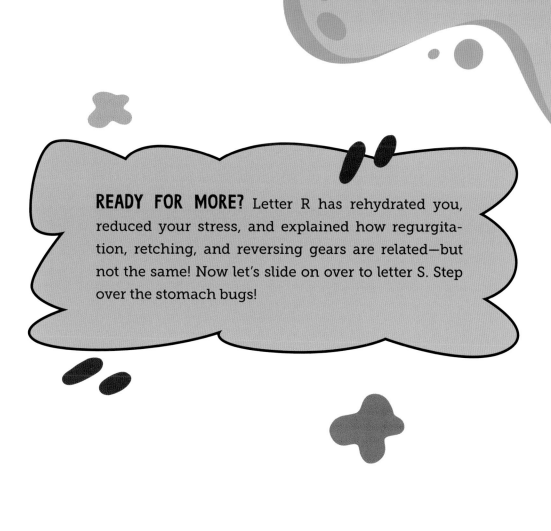

READY FOR MORE? Letter R has rehydrated you, reduced your stress, and explained how regurgitation, retching, and reversing gears are related—but not the same! Now let's slide on over to letter S. Step over the stomach bugs!

S

Ever **see stars** after you go on a spewing spree? Wonder what a **stomach bug** looks like? Feel like **shooting soup** when you see someone else doing it? Ever worried what would happen if you set lunch free in **space**? Stop wondering! Letter S even shares how to make **Splatcakes**!

TURN UP THE VOLUME ON YOUR
VOMIT VOCABULARY

Seasick: go for a boat ride and hurl over the side

Secondhand Dinner: see supper inside out

Set Lunch Free: open the gate and let the burger bolt ("Hey! Now that's fast food!")

Shoot Soup: slurp it all in and spout it all out

Sick: feel unwell, out of sorts, woozy, and green after eating an unclean tangerine

Sling Everything: fling a belly full

Slorge: what happens after you gorge and go all Curious George on bananas

Spewing Spree: feel sushi go splooshy

Spewnami: ride a rolling wave of vomit with an undercurrent of nausea

Spill the Soup: fill the potbelly with chowder, then move it out-er

Spit Up: receive a free sample of the slop to come

Surf the Wave: when you feel stoked, but the stomach feels provoked ("Dude! Hang loose! My gut wants to wipe out!")

CHUCK'S SICK SCIENCE

S Is for Stomach

Sure, the stomach holds the meals you munch, but that's not all. The gut comes stocked with digestive juices to break down your breakfast. That way, it's ready to slide on down to the small intestine, where the nutrients you need can be absorbed.

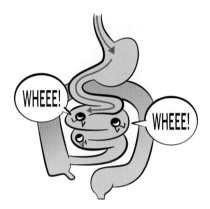

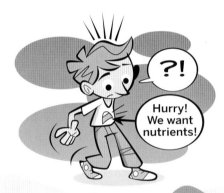

Queezy's Question

Why do I see stars when I "shoot soup"?

 PROFESSOR ANITA PUKE: Those are phosphenes.

 QUEEZY: I think "fuzz friends" are pretty.

 Phosphenes—or those "stars" you see—are caused by increased pressure on the eyes when you vomit. You might see phosphenes after a big sneeze or cough too.

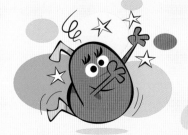

187

Queezy's Question

You sound sick. I mean, can a sound make me sick?

 PROFESSOR ANITA PUKE: More research is needed, but it is possible that high-frequency sounds could make some people feel dizzy and nauseous.

QUEEZY: A high-frequency sound? You mean you hear it frequently?

 It's called ultrasound. It's all around in the air, but the sound is too high for human ears to detect. Ultrasound can come from loudspeakers, door sensors, or machines for industrial cleaning or drilling.

If people can't hear the sound, how do we know that's what makes them sick?

 Researchers measured ultrasound in places where people complained about getting sick, such as railway stations, museums, schools, and sports stadiums. Factories where workers felt sick were studied too. Children and young adults were found to be more sensitive to the high-frequency sounds than adults.

I don't like the sound of that.

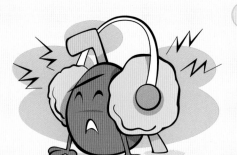

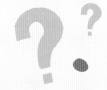

Emesis Etymology

WHERE DID THAT WORD COME FROM?

Bug (as in Stomach Bug)

By the eighteenth century, the word was related to bedbugs. (Bedbugs are actual insects and definitely pests. The old saying "Sleep tight! Don't let the bedbugs bite!" is no joke!)

Then, in the twentieth century, *bug* got connected to the tiny illness-causing microbes, or germs, that you can't see.

18TH CENTURY

20TH CENTURY

1622 ——————————————→ **TODAY**

The word *bug* was first used in 1622 to mean an imaginary scary thing.

19TH CENTURY

In the nineteenth century, the word *bug* referred to someone who can't let go of something, like an idea or asking for something they want.

So the way we use the word now— *stomach bug*—is really a combo of a "scary" thing you can't see that won't let go of you (at least not right away).

Queezy's Question

What does a stomach bug look like?

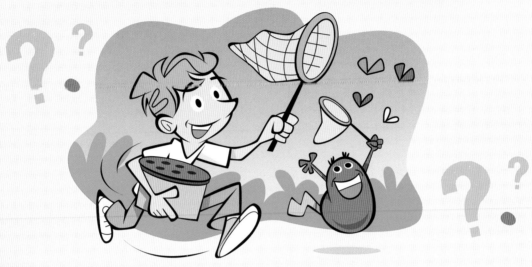

 PROFESSOR ANITA PUKE: What are you doing with that net?

QUEEZY: Chuck dared me to catch a stomach bug. No luck so far.

 I can assure you, there are no actual insects involved in what some call a stomach bug. The medical term is *viral gastroenteritis.* It is an infection in the intestine that is caused by a virus, resulting in stomach cramps, nausea, and vomiting. The most common way to "catch" gastroenteritis is from someone who already has the virus.

In that case, I'll wait and "catch" up with my friend after they get better.

 You're catching on!

Splatcakes

MAKES 8 SPLATCAKES

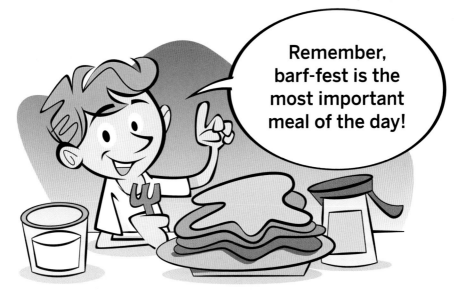

Remember, barf-fest is the most important meal of the day!

 Before you begin: Practice food safety (and avoid the vomit). Always start by washing your hands and cleaning the area of the kitchen where you'll be cooking. You'll want an adult to help you. Make sure your assistant has clean hands too!

YOU WILL NEED:

- 2 cups pancake batter mix
- 1 cup milk
- 2 eggs

HERE'S WHAT YOU NEED TO DO:

Step 1: Stir pancake mix, milk, and eggs in a bowl.

Step 2: Heat griddle or frying pan on medium-high.

Step 3: Pour ¼ cup of batter on hot griddle. Slide the flat edge of a spatula through the pancake while it's still wet. You want the edges of the pancakes to look like a splash instead of having smooth rounded edges.

TOPPINGS

• 2 cups applesauce mixed with crushed graham crackers

• 1 chopped apple and/ or banana

Step 4: When the edges of the splatcake look dry and there are bubbles in the center, flip it over. Cook that side about a minute. Use the spatula to move the splatcake to a plate.

Step 5: Spoon the toppings over each splatcake.

CHUCK'S SICK SCIENCE

Sympathetic Nervous System

PROFESSOR ANITA PUKE: When the stomach is ready to "unleash the monster," the sympathetic nervous system raises your heart rate and makes you perspire all over.

CHUCK: Isn't a spewing spree bad enough?

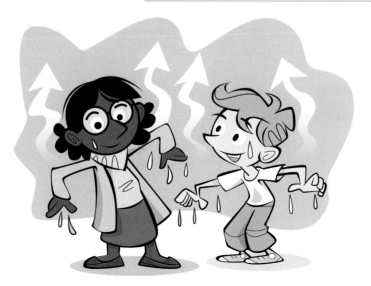

Sweating is helpful. The heat from your muscles is cooled as the sweat evaporates (begins to dry) across your body.

QUEEZY: See, Chuck? You have a built-in air conditioner!
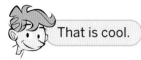

That is cool.

Queezy's Question

What happens if you launch animated throat missiles in space?

PROFESSOR ANITA PUKE: In other words, what happens when an astronaut vomits while in outer space?

QUEEZY: Puke-cisely!

Astronauts traveling to the International Space Station can get "space sick," or what NASA refers to as space adaptation syndrome. Imagine floating in the space station with hash browns hovering around in the stomach. If that floating food needs to blast out, you "spill the soup" in outer space. Due to the low gravity inside the space station, there would be—

CHUCK: Ka-BLAM! Astro-arf across the Milky Way!

Thankfully, astronauts have a bag to use for vomiting.

Like a barf bag on an airplane?

Almost. This is a special plastic bag lined with material to protect the face from floating vomit. When the astronaut stops vomiting, she can wipe her face on the liner, then push the liner into the bag and seal it up.

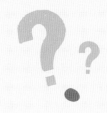 What does the astronaut do with that sack of atomic vomit?

 The used bag must be stored in the space station, maybe for months, while the crew is still in space.

 That is the worst souvenir ever.

 Can we make Puke Punch floats now?

Queezy's Question

Why do I feel like going on a spewing spree when I see someone gag or getting sick?

 PROFESSOR ANITA PUKE: Scientists aren't exactly sure why, but hearing or seeing someone vomit—even in a movie—can cause some people to feel nauseated, gag, or set their lunch free. It may be nature's way of protecting us from harmful food since prehistoric times. For some reason, it's stuck with us. So if you saw someone getting sick after eating a . . .

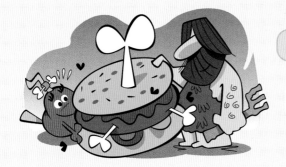

QUEEZY: Brachiosaurus burger!

. . . you'd look for something else to eat, wouldn't you?

Patagosaurus pizza? T. rex taco?

Thanks, Queezy. I'll take a nice green salad. Now, back to your question—besides providing possible prehistoric protection, feeling nauseated at the sight of someone else vomiting may be connected to a memory of the last time you spewed your splatcakes.

Hmm. That reminds me to ask if you have any syrup.

LETTER S sure didn't sell itself short. Did you see stars when you learned about spewing in space?

Ticket, please! Time to take a trip to letter T. Train travel used to be terrifying. Today it's typically not too much trouble until you get motion sickness. Look at what to do to get yourself back on track.

Let's take off!

T

Try not to worry after you read the part about the octopus in the **toilet.** Troubled by the thought of **teeth melting** if you **throw up**? (Queezy is too!) The terrible taste of **toilet yodel** can torture the tongue. Discover the source of that sour.

TURN UP THE VOLUME ON YOUR VOMIT VOCABULARY

Technicolor Yawn: open wide and let the rainbow flow to the bathroom bowl

Throw Up: after a cup of cheese soup, the gut winds up, then blows up . . . heads up!

Tip the Shopping Cart: when groceries roll up on the belly's conveyor belt

Toilet Yodel: overeat Swiss cheese and blow it out your yodel hole

Tonsil Toss: feel the loss of the applesauce as it shoots across the tonsils

Toss Your Tacos: when you hear lunch say "vamos" (let's go) and then it does ("Bye! Sad to see you go, tacos!")

Tummy Tantrum: when the belly blows up and tosses tofu in the toilet

625 BCE Rome—Home of the Kitchen Toilet and the Pantry Octopus

Romans were delighted to take over regions already fitted with a massive underground sewer system by the Etruscans. (The Etruscan culture covered a large portion of northwestern Italy, but after a series of wars with the Romans, their territory and society—along with their sewer system—became part of the Roman Empire.) As Roman cities grew, so did the piles of poo and pools of vomit (and other things that might make you want to, well, "toilet yodel"). Modern researchers believe that Romans used their sewer systems to drain water off their bumpy streets, but not the gross stuff floating on them.

The city of Pompeii had plenty of public toilets, but they weren't attached to the sewer either. Private homes had toilets (in the kitchen!), but those drained into a pit below the potty pipe.

Roman sewers had open pipes. Why not connect to a more sanitary system? Well, homeowners were more nervous about what might come up the pipes than about what they were putting down them. Researchers tell the story of a rich merchant who lived in a harbor city near Naples. Every night, a huge octopus swam from the sea and into the sewer, where it came up the man's toilet pipe to eat pickled fish in his pantry. Imagine bending over the toilet to throw up and finding an octopus staring back at you!

Queezy's Question

Can vomit melt your teeth?

PROFESSOR ANITA PUKE: Glands in the mouth create a watery fluid called saliva to help with tasting, chewing, and swallowing food. Saliva also keeps the mouth moist and starts the digestion of starches (which turn into sugars) in the food you eat. You produce enough saliva every day to fill almost six soda cans!

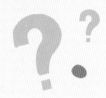

QUEEZY: Ew! That's enough to make me never drink soda again!

As for the teeth, the body makes extra saliva as it prepares for you to vomit. That saliva coats the teeth to protect them from stomach acid when you "splurge."

Aw. My body does that for me? My teeth get teensy spit coats.

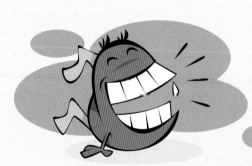

EVER HEARD of HYPERsalivation?
Slide on over to page 87
to read all about it.

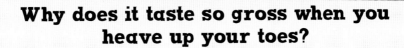

Queezy's Question

Why does it taste so gross when you heave up your toes?

PROFESSOR ANITA PUKE: Are you asking about the secret of vomit's signature sour stomach smoothie flavor?

CHUCK: You said a real mouth full there!

QUEEZY: Blech! I prefer a peppermint prune smoothie with a sprinkle of chopped onion.

You don't have to worry about me asking for a sip of that.

That's sweet.

You two are funny. Here's what's funny about stomach acid. It burns, but it's not sour or sweet. It's tasteless.

But vomit tastes so gross!

Vomit gets its disgusting flavor from butyl acid, a chemical made in the small intestine, combined with the digested and partly digested foods that were swirling together inside your body before you . . .

Toss your tacos!

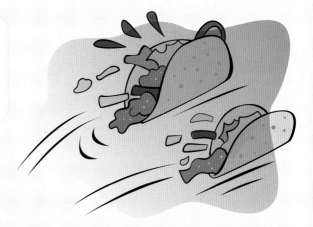

Queezy's Question

Why do my eyes tear up when I "tip the shopping cart"?

 PROFESSOR ANITA PUKE: You have different kinds of tears that do different jobs. Glands under the eyebrows push those tears out of the eyes when you need them.

QUEEZY: All my tears look the same to me.

 Irritant tears appear when you vomit to wash away things that may run or float into your eyes.

Vomiting does make me irritated.

QUEEZY'S FRIEND FIZZY SAYS

you can't toss your tonsils with your eyes open.
Is that true? Find out on page 58.

A Tale of Tongue Toads, Saliva Snakes, and a Gold Gush

Adapted from a French fairy tale

Once upon a time, there lived a woman with two daughters. She adored her older daughter, Crabgrass, because she was just like her—cranky, sour, and self-centered. The younger daughter, Lily, was kind and loving, but the other two despised her sweetness.

One day when Lily went to get water from the well, an old woman appeared asking for a drink. Good-hearted Lily was happy to help. Suddenly, the woman revealed herself to be a fairy. Impressed by Lily's gentle nature, the fairy gave her a reward. From then on, whenever Lily spoke, a jewel or gold would fall from her mouth.

As soon as Lily returned home, she told her mother about the fairy at the well. Dazzled by valuable surprises falling from Lily's lips, the greedy mother ordered Crabgrass to go to the well next. She couldn't wait to have twice the treasure!

When Crabgrass arrived at the well, a princess was waiting there. The princess politely asked for water, but the rude and jealous Crabgrass refused to help. It was then that the princess revealed herself to be a fairy. Disgusted by the disrespect Crabgrass had shown her, the fairy decided whenever Crabgrass uttered a sound, a snake or a toad would spill from her mouth.

Crabgrass trudged home to tell her mother the sad story. As she did, snakes and toads fell from her lips. The mother was furious. She blamed Lily for tricking them and ordered her to leave and never come back. Without a word, Lily walked to the door. The snakes and toads Crabgrass had spewed followed close behind. Little did the mother know the creatures had bellies full of Lily's gold and jewels, ready to return to her.

While alone in the woods, Lily met a prince as warmhearted as she was. In time, they married, and together they made a loving family of their own. Meanwhile, the grumpy mother became so repulsed by her snake-spewing, toad-lipped daughter, she kicked Crabgrass out too. Alone and poor, the snarly woman ate nothing but snake stew and lived crankily ever after.

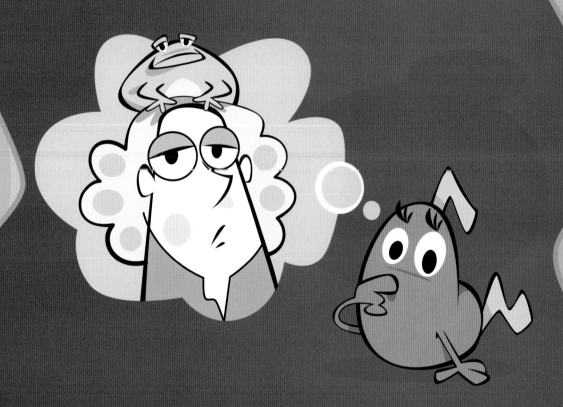

STAYING ON TRACK WITH TRAIN TRAVEL

Do people get motion sickness on a train?

The rocking motion of a train and the blur of scenery as you pass may put you on the track toward motion sickness. Try these tips to kick motion sickness in the caboose:

- **Sit near the front and stay seated.** Railway cars tend to have a steadier ride near the front of the train. The ideal spot would be a seat in the middle of the first car.

- **Face forward.** Instead of turning your head to look out the window, keep your head facing forward so you can see the scenery as it comes toward you.

- **Keep your cool.** The train may have fresh air vents near each seat that you can adjust as needed. Many trains are equipped with air conditioning too. You may want to bring a small personal fan and a few bottles of water in a backpack to stay cool and hydrated.

HURLED HISTORY

Rough Way to Ride the Rails

Early Days of Railway Travel

In the 1800s, before the automobile (and car sickness) existed, people relied on trains for transportation. Passengers on the swaying trains often suffered from "railway sickness."

Motion sickness medicine did not exist in the early 1800s, so to avoid railway sickness, some people thought it helped to carry a potato in their suitcase or to stuff newspaper under their shirt. Those ideas sound silly, but to be fair, rail travel really was dangerous in those days. Accidents were common. Passengers had reason to want some comfort.

Doctors called the panic and anxiety caused by motion sickness "railway shock." No wonder some passengers needed to "toilet yodel" or "choo choo spew spew" on the train.

QUEEZY: Too bad they couldn't look at page 205 to get them back on track.

TEARY EYES, melting teeth, toilet tentacles, and terrifying train travel? And what about the toad tongues? Hope letter T didn't leave a terrible taste in your mouth.

Up ahead is the unique letter U. You'll be introduced to the unusual tale of Ukemochi, who lets his utterly unrestrained creativity flow far and wide. It's unbelievable!

(Hey, you think you're the only one with a uvula? U R about to find out!)

U

Under the weather today? Uncover where that expression came from. Upgrade simple spuds with a new **Unleash the Monster Mash** recipe. Find out how to clean **upholstery** after you **upchuck.** Then you'll meet the unusual **uvula** too. It may make your jaw unhinged!

TURN UP THE VOLUME ON YOUR VOMIT VOCABULARY

Uncap the Queso: send the spicy nachos on a trip

Un-Food: feel food in your stomach dash for the nearest exit

Unleash the Monster: spew an ogre out of your innards

Unpack: come home from camp and drop a load of dirty socks

Up and Out: when the food that's been down-and-in celebrates Opposite Day ("I wish my dinner did the opposite!")

Upchuck: muck out the yuck that's stuck in the middle

Urp: the surprise of a burp with a bonus

Unleash the Monster Mash

`- - - - - - - - - - - ->` **MAKES 4 SERVINGS**

YOU WILL NEED:

- 1 cup instant mashed potato flakes
- 1/3 cup milk (or milk substitute)
- 2 tablespoons butter
- 1 small can (10.5–12 oz.) peas and carrots (drain off water)
- 1 small can (10.5–12 oz.) corn (drain off water)
- 1 drop each of red and yellow food coloring (to make orange)
- Salt and pepper

⭐ *Before you begin:* Practice food safety (and avoid the vomit). Always start by washing your hands and cleaning the area of the kitchen where you'll be cooking. You'll want an adult to help you. Make sure your assistant has clean hands too!

HERE'S WHAT YOU NEED TO DO:

Step 1: Follow directions on instant mashed potato box, which will be something like this:

- Put 1⅔ cups of water and 2 tablespoons of butter in a saucepan, and bring to a boil over medium-high heat.

- As soon you see bubbles, take the pan off the heat. Pour in the milk and the potato flakes. Stir. Then wait about a minute for the potatoes to thicken.

- Add one drop of red food coloring and one drop of yellow. Stir.

Step 2: Dump the rest of the ingredients into the prepared potatoes. Give it a stir.

UPHOLSTERY—HOW TO CLEAN IF YOU BARF IN THE BACKSEAT

Okay, so you "uncapped the queso" on the upholstery of Professor Puke's vehicle. It happens. Here's what you need to do:

Step 1: Put on rubber gloves for safety, then scrape up the big chunks with a spatula or a thick paper towel.

Step 2: Blot the wetness with a paper towel.

Step 3: Sprinkle baking soda over the area to help remove vomit odor. Wait 30 minutes. Use a cordless vacuum if there's one available.

Step 4: Toss the paper towels and rubber gloves in a covered trash container to avoid spreading germs. Wash your hands.

IF CAR RIDES cause you to "uncap the queso,"
go to page 38 to make a pre-ride plan.

**FOR UNCLE URP'S 5½ TIPS FOR
CLEANING UP CARPET COLLYWOBBLES,**
go to page 39.

ICKY IDIOMS

Under the Weather

When someone is "under the weather," it means they don't feel well. If you've ever had to "unleash the sea monster," you know what being under the weather feels like.

What's the connection between weather and the urge to upchuck? Sea travelers aboard a ship battling rough waves and wind would head belowdecks to try to avoid seasickness. Tucked inside their cabins, they were "under the weather."

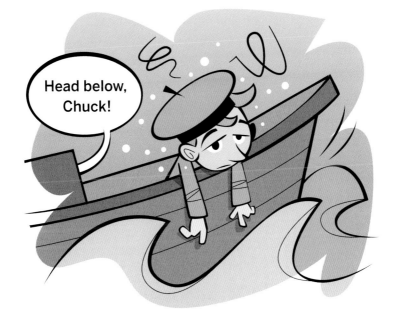

WAS THAT the best way (or place) to go on a boat?
Sail on over to page 130 to find out.

CHUCK'S SICK SCIENCE

U Is for Uvula

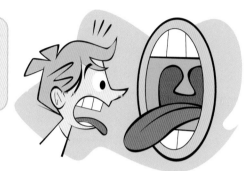

CHUCK: Go get a mirror. Open wide. Say AHHHHH. Look way in the back of your mouth. See that thing that looks like a little punching bag hanging over your tongue? That's your uvula.

The uvula is part of the soft palate and moves backward so what you eat and drink doesn't go up your nose when you swallow. It also squirts out saliva (spit) to keep the mouth and throat from feeling dry.

TRUE OR FALSE?

Humans are the only ones who have a uvula.

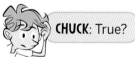
CHUCK: True?

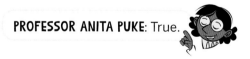
PROFESSOR ANITA PUKE: True.

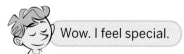
Wow. I feel special.

Ukemochi, the Grain–Gushing Japanese Goddess

The *Nihongi* (*The Chronicles of Japan*) tells the story of the goddess Ukemochi, who vomits fruit, vegetables, and fish into the world. Her puke even results in the creation of day and night.

The Sun, known as Amaterasu, sends her brother—the Moon—to visit Ukemochi. To welcome the Moon, Ukemochi vomits a flood of food on the table. The Moon finds this so disgusting that he draws his sword and kills Ukemochi in her own dining room.

But that doesn't put an end to Ukemochi's ability to produce food. Out from her lifeless mouth pours beans, and millet (grain) comes from her eyes. In Japan, it is said that rice is the soul, and the belly is where the soul lives. It's no surprise then that rice came out of Ukemochi's belly as a parting gift.

IT'S UNANIMOUS! You understand your uvula. How could you ever feel under the weather again now that you know how to use utensils to make Unleash the Monster Mash?

You're on the verge of letter V! Get ready to visualize a vomiting machine and visit a vomiting center. Venture on to letter V!

V

Letter V is no vacation! It's like a vortex whirling with vast, varied, and verifiable facts and figures. For example: 25,000! That's how many **villi** you have in every square inch of your small intestine. What are villi? Don't be silly. Let's venture on! A **vomitorium** and a **Vomit Comet** are in view!

TURN UP THE VOLUME ON YOUR
VOMIT VOCABULARY

Vaulting Vittles: when what's in your middle leaps over the tongue

Vent Gross Grub: release greasy gobs from your belly blobs

Vile Veggie Vacation: produce a glistening pool of broccoli, beets, and tomato juice

Visit Barfville: drop by the world's grossest rest stop and leave a souvenir

Vombination Unlock: when your body uses the right combination to empty the vault

Vombo Combo: when peanut butter and jelly from the deli mix with pickles in the belly ("Who ordered takeout?")

Vomcano: expel lunch-ish-looking lava from your mouth

Vomit: drop the waffles off at the whirlpool ("Whee!")

Voomerang: when you finish a snack only to have it come back around

INTRODUCING VILLI, THE CELL-COVERED STRAWS OF THE SMALL INTESTINE

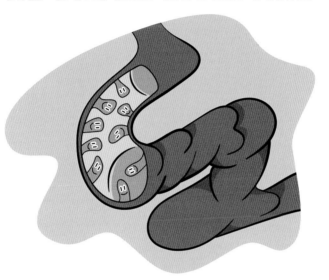

Job number one for the small intestine is to soak up nutrients from the chyme (partly digested food and stomach acid) passing by. Villi look like little fingers on the inside of the small intestines. They're like tiny cell-covered spongy straws slurping up the healthy stuff so it can be shipped to the rest of the body.

 QUEEZY: They sound adorable. I wish I could have a pet villus. It could play with Lickety Split!

 PROFESSOR ANITA PUKE: Then you'll be happy to hear this! You already have up to 25,000 villi per square inch (or up to 40 per square millimeter) of the small intestine.

 Wow! I better eat more fruits and veggies to feed my litter of villi.

Emesis Etymology

(WHERE DID THAT WORD COME FROM?)

Villi (plural), or Villus (singular)

The Latin word *villus* means "shaggy haired," like an animal with a long, hairy coat. But when Italian anatomist Gabriele Falloppio first used the word in his *Observationes anatomicae,* published in 1561, he described villi as having the texture of velvet. The inside of the intestinal wall does look velvety. But today, with the help of modern microscopes, we know that the "velvet" is made of tiny fingerlike projections of villi.

TAKE TIME TO LEARN ABOUT CHYME,
the favorite snack of villi. See page 43.

HURLED HISTORY

Professor Anita Puke Busts the Myth of the Vomitorium

 PROFESSOR ANITA PUKE: Ah! I do love to bust a myth.

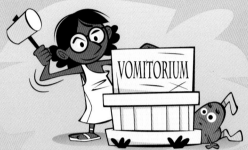

Let's start with the word *vomitorium,* because that is where the confusion starts. The Latin root for the word *vomitorium* does mean "to spew forth." But it does not refer to vomiting. The myth goes that rich citizens of Rome would host huge feasts where their guests would stuff themselves with exotic foods and then head to a place called a vomitorium to "vault vittles," as Queezy might say.

Here's the real story: A Roman writer named Macrobius used the term *vomitoria* (meaning more than one vomitorium) in his book *Saturnalia* in the fifth century CE. He was writing about a passageway in a theater where Roman citizens would go to watch a play. These passages were wide enough for many theatergoers to enter, or make a fast exit in case of a fire. So people would "spew forth" by walking through the vomitorium.

However, ancient Roman history experts also say guests at a big banquet bash would go to a room near the dining hall, not a place called a vomitorium, to barf after gorging on platters of goodies. This made room for more fancy food like stuffed dormouse or parrot tongue fricassee. Classy.

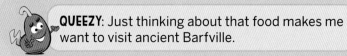 **QUEEZY:** Just thinking about that food makes me want to visit ancient Barfville.

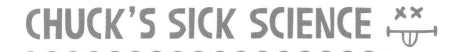

CHUCK'S SICK SCIENCE

Virus

A tiny organism that is only seen with a microscope. It invades living cells and spreads sickness. Here's an example:

Viral Gastritis

An infection in the belly from a stomach virus. It's commonly called the stomach flu.

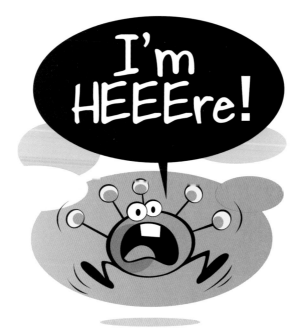

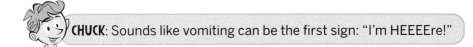

CHUCK: Sounds like vomiting can be the first sign: "I'm HEEEEre!"

Queezy's Question

What is the Vomit Comet?

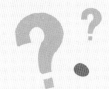

PROFESSOR ANITA PUKE: In 1957, the National Aeronautics and Space Administration (NASA) space shuttle crew had a tough time with motion sickness. So a Boeing transport aircraft was converted into a reduced-gravity aircraft called the KC-135 that would help astronauts get used to the feeling of zero-gravity spaceflight.

QUEEZY: You mean it was like they were floating in outer space?

Spot on! The high-flying aircraft would climb up to 34,000 feet to give trainees about thirty seconds of weightlessness. The feeling was like a skydiving free fall. In a three-hour NASA training mission, there could be forty of these powerful up-and-down trips. All the roller-coastery climbing and diving made astronauts sick. That's how the aircraft got its unofficial nickname of the Vomit Comet. It was also called the Barf Buzzard.

I'll take the bus. Thanks.

CHUCK'S SICK SCIENCE

Welcome to the Vomiting Center

A vomcano takes coordination. It starts with a signal to the brain's vomiting center. Then the vomiting center sends an alert when it's time to go into action.

The vomiting center is an exciting place to hang out in your brain. Get more details on page 81.

EVER SEEN A VOMITING MACHINE?

Dr. Lee-Ann Jaykus, a professor at North Carolina State University, had a hunch that when a person with norovirus throws up, tiny norovirus particles are aerosolized. That means the virus becomes a fine spray that floats through the air and can pass to other people. To put her hunch to the test, Dr. Jaykus and her team decided to build a vomiting machine.

In 2014, they filled the machine's "belly" with fake vomit made of pudding mixed with a less dangerous form of the virus. Then, for safety, the machine was locked in a large clear box. When the machine "vomited," up to 10,000 virus particles flew into the air. And it only takes twenty particles to infect someone. Dr. Jaykus's hunch was correct!

CHECK OUT page 166 for more on flying fast food.

MEET THE VAGUS NERVE

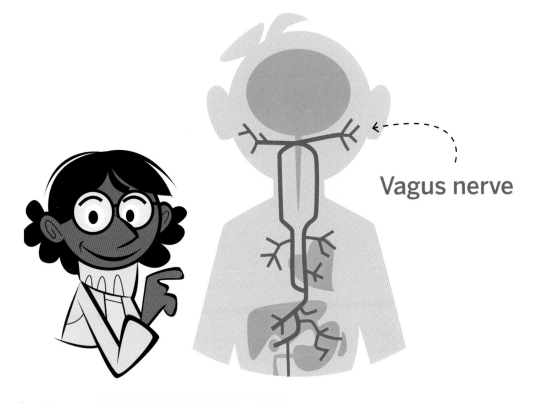

Vagus nerve

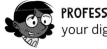 **PROFESSOR ANITA PUKE**: Do you know what is managing your digestive tract right this very moment?

QUEEZY: I don't have the "vagus" idea.

 Queezy! It sounds like you do! The vagus nerve, which is actually a set of nerves, starts in the brain stem at the base of the skull and then branches out from there to do its many jobs. For example, the vagus nerve controls the muscles throughout the body's digestive system so that the stomach muscles know when to push food to the digestive tract and so much more.

I'd like to see the manager, please!

VAST AMOUNTS of valuable information were found in the letter V vault. Professor Puke valiantly unveiled the truth behind the vomitorium myth. Very interesting.

Well, let's wander over to letter W. Wait until you read the part about whales, an egg-loving king, and a worthwhile way to unwind when you may need to "whistle chunks." And watch for the part where we wonder no more about the reason *why* we vomit in the first place! (It's quite wise.)

W

Welcome to letter W, where we'll wonder about **word vomit** and . . .

Whoa! Wait! **Why do we vomit?** Why would we worry about **whale vomit** and what a wealthy ruler had for breakfast? That's silly. And **wash our hands**? Why? Whales only have flippers. That reminds me, where are my slippers? Who am I talking to? What does it matter? Oooh. Matter rhymes with back splatter, like at the end of this book. I'm in a book?! That's wonderful!

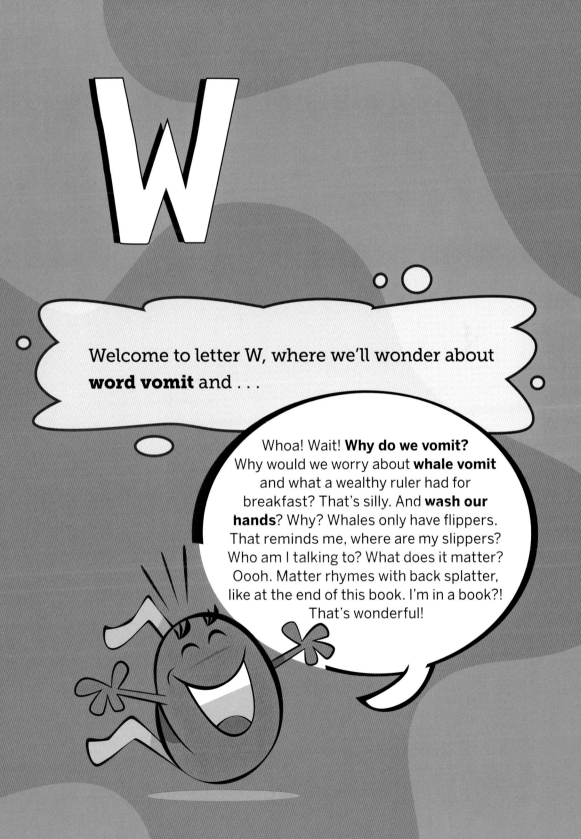

TURN UP THE VOLUME ON YOUR VOMIT VOCABULARY

Waah: hurl so hard you make your stomach sob

Waves of Woe: vomit not once but repeatedly, while sailing stormy seas ("Abandon ship!")

Wear Your Lunch: what happens when vomit makes you a whole new outfit

Wet Burp: learn what an inside-out wet burrito looks like ("Dude. I cannot unsee that.")

Whistle Chunks: blow barf for all to hear

Whoa: Hold on to the sink! What's that pink stink? ("Did you eat the whole watermelon?")

Whoopsie: when you aim for the bowl but miss the whole hole

Woop: slip out a sloppy scoop of goopy gut soup, as in "Oops. I wooped my boots."

Queezy's Question

Is "word vomit" a real thing?

CHUCK: Professor Puke, let me handle this one. Word vomit happens when you say out loud all the words that are swirling around in the whirlpool that is your brain.

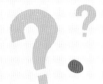

I wonder if Chuck knows he smells like burnt popcorn, mustard, and wet gym socks.

Oopsie. Did I say that out loud? Wow. I hope my mouth is on mute.

Chuck's cat Donut ate my homework. Then Donut hurled in Chuck's backpack and his beagle named Bagel ate the hurl.

I told our teacher Chuck did it. Mmm. Now I want a bagel. But not burnt popcorn. Maybe mustard.

Yes, word vomit is a real thing.

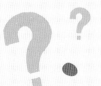

PROFESSOR ANITA PUKE: So I hear.

WASH YOUR HANDS

It's your sudsy superpower!

5 STEPS FOR HAND WASHING (ONE STEP FOR EACH FINGER)

Step 1: Get your hands wet under running water. Turn off the tap to save water.

Step 2: Grab the soap and rub your hands together. Suds up the backs of your hands and between your fingers. Clean under your nails too. Germs love to hang out there.

Step 3: Keep washing for twenty seconds or for as long as it takes you to say "ralphabet" 20 times.

Step 4: Rinse your hands well to wash away the soap and germs.

Step 5: Wipe your hands with a clean towel or let them air-dry. Don't skip this step! It's easier to spread germs with wet hands.

CHUCK'S SICK SCIENCE

Who Would Want to Wear Whale Puke (or Poop?) for Perfume?

 CHUCK: I'm not sure if this is made up or for real. Do you know anything about whale puke that's put in perfume?

PROFESSOR ANITA PUKE: You're thinking of ambergris. It's a waxy substance that can form in the gut of a sperm whale.

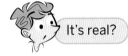 It's real?

Freshly expelled ambergris smells like feces.

 So, sperm whale poo?

At one point in history, ambergris was believed to be vomited up by whales. But those who find fresh ambergris say it is more likely poo than spew, based on its smell. Although it probably comes out of the whale's body like feces, ambergris is something else entirely.

 Hold on. How does it get in the whale's body? Where do you find it once it comes out?

For hundreds of years, it was assumed sperm whales ate something and then vomited it out. There were theories about the whale eating tree sap, sea-foam, or fungus. We now know it's made within the bile duct of the whale itself.

What? Then how do people find it?

Ambergris is washed ashore on beaches in parts of the world where sperm whales live. Because it's so rare, ambergris may be sold for more than silver or gold. In the summer of 2023, an animal health researcher in the Canary Islands came upon a dead sperm whale on the shore. Inside the whale was a chunk of ambergris weighing more than 20 pounds (9.5 kg). It was worth about $550,000. He hoped to sell it and donate the money to victims of a volcanic eruption on the island.

I'm still not sure I want to visit those beaches!

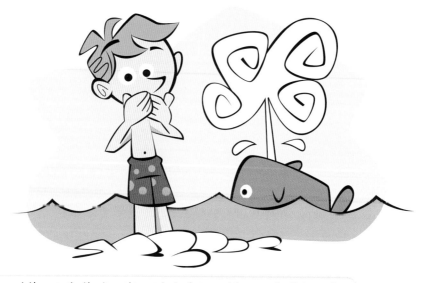

A recent theory is that ambergris is formed from a buildup of squid beaks that get stuck in the whale's intestine. The whale's fecal matter forms around it and creates a large blockage that eventually causes the intestine to burst, setting the ambergris free. Unfortunately, this kills the whale.

After it dries and ages in the open air and sunshine, the scent is described as musky (a warm, sweet smell), like pipe tobacco, or like the ocean. Makers of expensive perfumes add it to fragrances because it makes the other ingredients smell even better. Scientists created a version of ambergris in a lab, but it's not quite the same.

A Scrambled Case of Two Kings Named Charles and Ambergris

Over the centuries, ambergris was used in medicine. Containers of ambergris were tied around the waist to ward off the deadly bubonic plague. (Umm, in case you're wondering, it didn't work so well.)

Ambergris was added as an extra-special ingredient in one of the world's first recipes for ice cream. It even found its way into royal recipes! King Charles II of England was known to enjoy eggs and ambergris as his favorite meal.

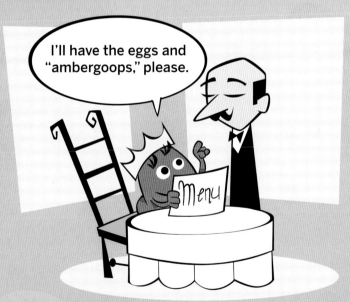

I'll have the eggs and "ambergoops," please.

But when King Charles II died unexpectedly, royal doctors suspected the king had been poisoned. In trying to crack the case, some wondered if the scent and flavor of the ambergris in his eggs could have concealed poison.

Modern scientists now guess the real cause of the king's death may be linked to his enjoyment of experimenting with mercury (a highly toxic element). Inhaling mercury vapors can cause nausea and vomiting and, in extreme cases, death. In the king's case, it's possible too much time in the royal basement laboratory was truly too much for him.

Fast-Forward 338 Years . . .

The coronation of King Charles III of England took place in May 2023. Unlike monarchs before him, King Charles III opted not to have ambergris (or other products from animals) added to the special oil used during his coronation ceremony. The aim was to be cruelty-free to animals.

Queezy's Question

Tell me again—WHY?! Why do we vomit?

 PROFESSOR ANITA PUKE. Our bodies do astounding things for us.

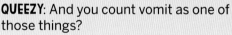 **QUEEZY:** And you count vomit as one of those things?

 I do. I would never call vomiting a fun experience. But it is far better than having something harmful pass through your whole digestive system. The human body is filled with sensors and systems designed to defend us. For example, your body causes you to sneeze to protect your nose and your lungs, and your eyes blink automatically to protect your eyes. Oftentimes, your body goes into action before you even know there's a problem. And that's what the ability to vomit does for you.

It's like having a home security system for the body.

See why I'm so passionate about puke?

Wow. Who knew puking protects me?

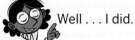

Well . . . I did.

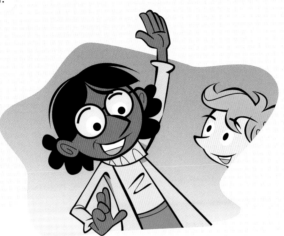

WORTH THE "WRIST"!

Put a Little Pressure on Yourself

Putting pressure on precise areas of the body may help you feel better. Try this to reduce nausea:

Step 1: With your palm facing you, put your index (pointer) finger, middle finger, and ring finger close together and place them across your arm, near the base of your palm/wrist.

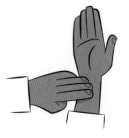

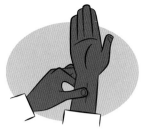

Step 2: Let your thumb go around so it's near the base of your hand/wrist on the other side.

Step 3: Use your thumb to rub this area using pressure and move it in a circular motion for three minutes.

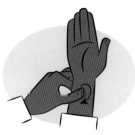

Step 4: Give your other wrist attention too.

Queezy's Question

WHAT?!
What happens in my body when I vomit?

WELCOME TO THE BARF BALLET

?

• The chemoreceptor trigger zone (CTZ) in the brain gets a message: "Tummy trouble!"

• Vomiting center in the brain sounds the alarm.

• Mouth makes extra saliva to protect itself and teeth from stomach acid.

• Lungs take a deep breath to keep from getting vomit in them.

• Diaphragm contracts (tightens) with a few short pulses, *squeeeezing* the stomach to create pressure.

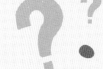

- Glottis closes to make sure nothing gets into the lungs.

- Abdominal muscles tighten for even more pressure.

- Pyloric sphincter (the one that opens to let food go into the small intestine) slams shut.

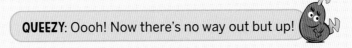

QUEEZY: Oooh! Now there's no way out but up!

- Sympathetic nervous system raises the heart rate and produces sweat to keep you cool.

WELL, WELL, WELL. We went from word vomit to whale "vomit" to why we vomit. Wow! We whooped out a wide range of weird and wondrous information.

There's more on the way. Why wait? Letter X has the scoop on xigua. What's xigua? You'd better X-it this page to find out!

X

Ready for a juicy slice of **xigua**? Not sure? How about trying it? But first, pay attention to how much is too much! Feeling anXious about a stomach **X-ray**? X-amine the truth so you can X-hale.

TURN UP THE VOLUME ON YOUR VOMIT VOCABULARY

Xanthic Banana Barf: produce pale, yellowish split-up scented with banana

X-It Up: send chewed food, which was once down, up and out again

X Marks the Spot: find the perfect place to puke

X-plosive Exports: push peppery puke out the mouth port

X-treme Emesis: vomit so hard, so loud, and so long that you'll tell the grandchildren about it one day

X IS FOR XIGUA

Xigua (SHE-gua) is the Chinese word for *watermelon.* Foods like xigua, as well as tomatoes and papayas, contain lycopene. Lycopene is a red pigment that gives xigua its rosy color. Scientists believe eating a balanced diet that includes *healthy* levels of lycopene may lower the risk of illnesses like heart disease or asthma, and even some kinds of cancer.

How Much Xigua Is Too Much of a Good Thing?

Eating more than 30 mg of lycopene-rich fruit like xigua can cause nausea and vomiting.

1½ cups of watermelon contains about 10 mg of lycopene.

Do the Math

If you eat more than 4½ cups of xigua in one sitting, you likely won't be sitting long. That's like eating three pounds of watermelon cubes! You'll be running to the bathroom to "X-It Up" all that juicy xigua!

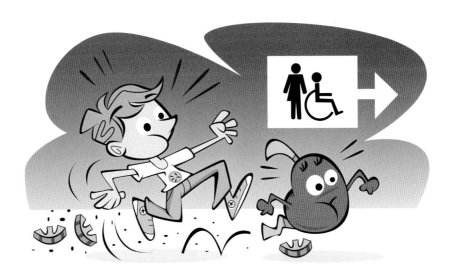

Queezy's Question

Can getting an X-ray cause X-plosive exports?

PROFESSOR ANITA PUKE: No. An X-ray of the stomach area won't make you puke, but it may help the doctor figure out the cause of belly pain or vomiting. What shows up on a stomach X-ray? Images could include a kidney stone, a hole or blockage in the intestine, or even a "what is that?!" you accidentally swallowed.

QUEEZY: Could the doctor see the xigua seeds I swallowed?

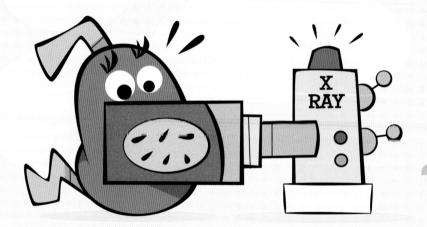

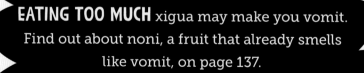

EATING TOO MUCH xigua may make you vomit.
Find out about noni, a fruit that already smells
like vomit, on page 137.

YOU LEARNED another word for watermelon—*xigua*—and how much melon is too much if you want to avoid making X-plosive exports. (Of course you do!) Plus, you got the good news that X-rays won't make you X-pel the bacon and eggs.

Let's X-it letter X and yield to letter Y because "Y" not? You're about to learn the truth about yellow yurk. And, yes, you'll also find out what to eat after you make it. Yum?

Y

Yikes! **Yellow yeech** can make you screech. But how does that color come up? Yearning for a snack to help your belly feel better? You'll say "yeah!" to a soothing smoothie recipe and yummy yogurt treat.

TURN UP THE VOLUME ON YOUR VOMIT VOCABULARY

Yack Your Snack: return a liquefied lunch into your backpack

Yarf: explode the whole of it, not the harf (half) of it

Yawp: cry for yelp (help) after slurping down kelp

Yeech: hawk up a peach—pit and all—on the beach

Yell at the Ground: shout slop at the floor

Yodel Your Lunch: set the cheesy fondue free in Switzerland ("Ew. My song came out wrong!")

Yo-Yo: what goes down . . . may come up . . . then down (and all over!)

Yuck: disgust even yourself

Yurk: go berserk and hurl a ham on rye at your homework ("Sorry, Ms. Snard. I yurked on my work.")

Queezy's Question

What makes my yurk yellow?

PROFESSOR ANITA PUKE: Blame bile. Yellow or greenish-yellow yurk is due to a fluid called bile. The liver is the bile maker, and the gallbladder stores it for you.

QUEEZY: That's so sweet, Ms. Gall Bladder. You're my kind of "gall."

Yurking on an empty belly makes bile more likely to appear. Bile may be a gross color, but it has important jobs to do. For example, bile helps the body soak up vitamins, and it removes waste from the body, such as used red blood cells.

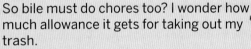
So bile must do chores too? I wonder how much allowance it gets for taking out my trash.

Bile also breaks down the fats in food you eat so the body can use them for energy.

Oooh. Like a triple-decker cheeseburger.

It sounds to me like it gets paid in cheeseburgers.

Aha! That's how it gets its cheesy, mustardy color!

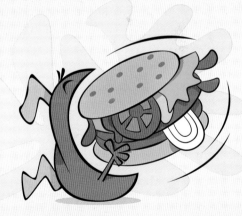

CHECK OUT Chuck's Coloring Book of Chunk for more color combos on page 41.

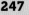

Yeech on the Beach

The perfect post-yack snack!

MAKES 1 SERVING

YOU WILL NEED:

- ½ cup graham cracker crumbs
- 1 single serving of yogurt (any flavor or even plain, but a runny variety works best for this recipe)

Queezy's Tip

After you're sure you've had your last yack, choose soft, bland (not spicy) foods, like yogurt, to help you get your strength back and get your gut in good shape again.

⭐ **Before you begin:** Practice food safety (and avoid the vomit). Always start by washing your hands and cleaning the area of the kitchen where you'll be cooking. You'll want an adult to help you. Make sure your assistant has clean hands too!

HERE'S WHAT YOU NEED TO DO:

Step 1: Sprinkle graham cracker crumbs into a cereal bowl or short drinking glass. (Think of the crumbs like a sandy beach.)

Step 2: Pour or scoop yogurt on top of the "sand."

Step 3: If you want "shells" on the beach, you could add a *few* yogurt-covered raisins.

Queezy's Tip

Don't gulp it down. Go slow. Don't feel like eating it all at once? That's okay. Keep leftovers covered and cool in the refrigerator until you're ready to hit the beach again.

Yogurt Spewthie

Try a spewthie for breakfast the next day to boost the energy.

MAKES 2 SERVINGS

YOU WILL NEED:

• 1 cup apple juice (once you feel 100 percent better, you can use other juices)

• 1 cup plain or vanilla Greek yogurt

• 1 cup frozen fruit

• 1 cup spinach

• 2 cups ice cubes

⭐ **Before you begin:** Practice food safety (and avoid the vomit). Always start by washing your hands and cleaning the area of the kitchen where you'll be cooking. You'll want an adult to help you. Make sure your assistant has clean hands too!

HERE'S WHAT YOU NEED TO DO:

Step 1: Pour juice into the blender.

Step 2: Dump in the yogurt, frozen fruit, and spinach.

Step 3: Pop the lid on the blender and mix a minute or so until smooth.

Step 4: Add 1 cup of ice and blend. Remove lid and check to see if the smoothie looks the way you like it. Is it too thick? Add up to one more cup of ice.

Step 5: Pour into two tall glasses. Slip in a straw. Go slow! Slurp like a sleepy snail.

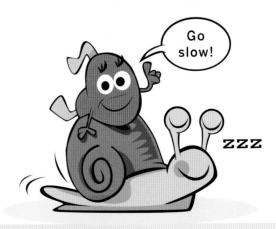

Go slow!

zzz

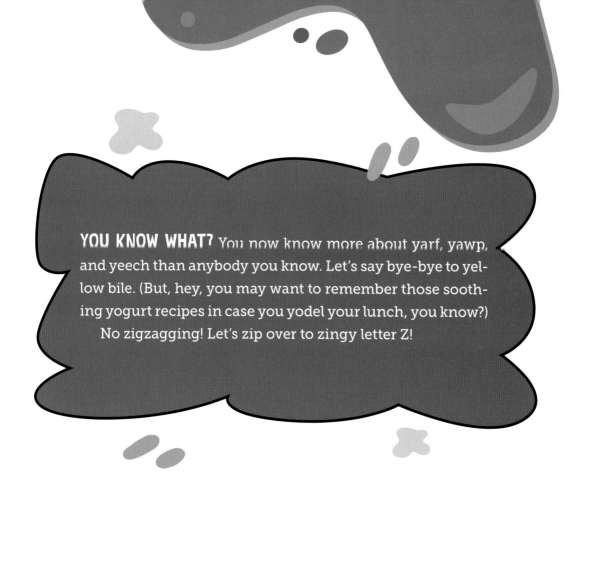

YOU KNOW WHAT? You now know more about yarf, yawp, and yeech than anybody you know. Let's say bye-bye to yellow bile. (But, hey, you may want to remember those soothing yogurt recipes in case you yodel your lunch, you know?) No zigzagging! Let's zip over to zingy letter Z!

Z

Zowie! We've reached "**Z**" end!

Don't zonk out yet! Find out what to do before you let **zinc** sink into the belly. It may sound zany, but what's the deal with the mutating **zucchini**? How do you eat 'em or zap 'em? Learn the best thing to do when there's zilch—no more **zoo spew** to spew too.

TURN UP THE VOLUME ON YOUR VOMIT VOCABULARY

Zilch: spew until there's zero left in your stomach

Zink: empty the contents of your stomach in the kitchen ("I had to zink in the sink.")

Zombie Zarf: barf your brains out

Zool: hurl into a body of water ("I had to zool in the pool.")

Zoo Spew: when the vomit smells like petting zoo poo

Zork: drop your fork and let your fish sticks fly

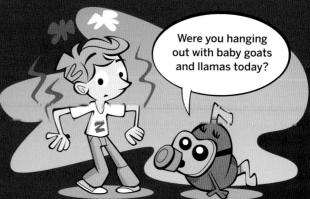

Were you hanging out with baby goats and llamas today?

Zowerswop: sip so much zippy zuppa, it comes back uppa

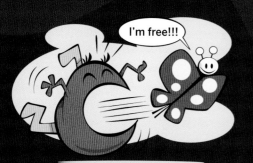

I'm free!!!

Zuke: puke for the last time (that day), as in "My belly is zuked out."

Zutter: accidentally inhale a butterfly and barf it up

CHUCK'S SICK SCIENCE

Z Is for Zinc

 PROFESSOR ANITA PUKE: Zinc is a mineral that can do all kinds of good things for the body. It can help you heal, grow, see, and a whole lot more. The thing is, the body doesn't have a zinc bank.

CHUCK: If there's no bank, how do I make a "deposit"?

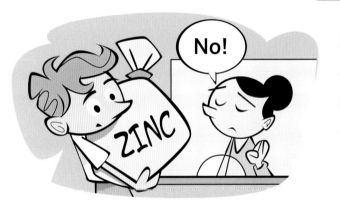

No!

The body counts on you to eat foods like meat, chicken, fish, tofu, and whole-grain cereal to get the zinc it needs. If you can't add zinc that way, the doctor may want you to take a zinc tablet each day.

 Sounds smart, but what's all this got to do with vomit?

If you swallow a zinc tablet without eating something first, your empty gut can get annoyed. The more that tablet breaks down, the more your belly complains. And you know what that means!

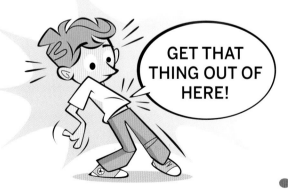

GET THAT THING OUT OF HERE!

ZOWIE!

When mutant squash run wild, or the case of toxic zucchini syndrome

Meet the cucurbits family. This friendly bunch of "melon heads" includes gourds like pumpkins and zucchini squash. Most of the time, these are mild, tasty, healthy vegetables you can grow in a home garden or find at a farm market.

It hardly ever happens, but in certain situations, zucchini can cause toxic squash syndrome. That's when the squash mingles with a wild plant and mutates. The wild plant produces a chemical called cucurbitacins [CUE-kur-bih-tay-sins] to protect itself against insects. Wonderful for the wild plant, but horrible for humans.

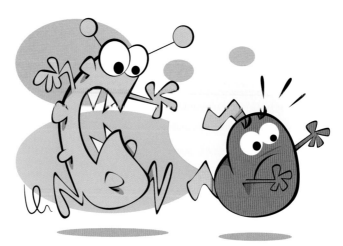

An easy way to know if you have a problem plant is to do a taste test. Slice the top off the zucchini and touch your tongue to it. If it's extremely bitter, trust your tongue and squash that squash. If you were to eat a few bites, you could end up with belly cramps, dizziness, nausea, and vomiting.

Queezy's Last Question

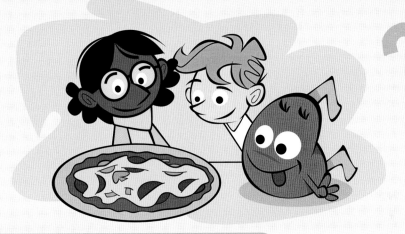

 CHUCK: What?! We've reached the end already?

 QUEEZY: Hey, speaking of "end," what should I do after my body stops zorking?

 PROFESSOR ANITA PUKE: Vomiting can feel like a lot of work. Once it's done, sit in a room that's quiet and calm. Count to five while taking deep breaths. Drink a few sips of water. Lie down if you want, but sit up before sipping more water.

 Slurp-slurp-slurp.

 Oh! And stay away from heavy, greasy foods like pizza or spaghetti, and bubbly drinks like soda. Let your belly take a break.

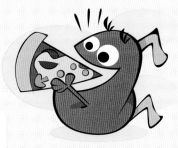

 Thanks, Professor Puke!

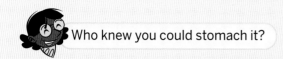 Who knew you could stomach it?

 All this talk about puke is making me hungry. Can we go feed our faces now?

 I need to go feed the fishes again! But when I come back, I want a bagel topped with mint jelly, sardines, candy corn, and radishes.

GO TO page 248 for a soothing post-yack snack recipe.

CONGRATULATIONS!
YOU ARE NOW A VERIFIED
VOMITOLOGIST!

Who knows more about spew than you do?
(Other than Professor Anita Puke, of course!)
 And now you know there's so much more to
know than you ever knew there was to know.
 Take good care of your unbelievable body.
It sure tries to take care of you and protect you
even when—*especially when*—you need to "yell
at your shoes."

YOU DESERVE A BARFTASTIC BONUS!
Check out the Back Splatter!

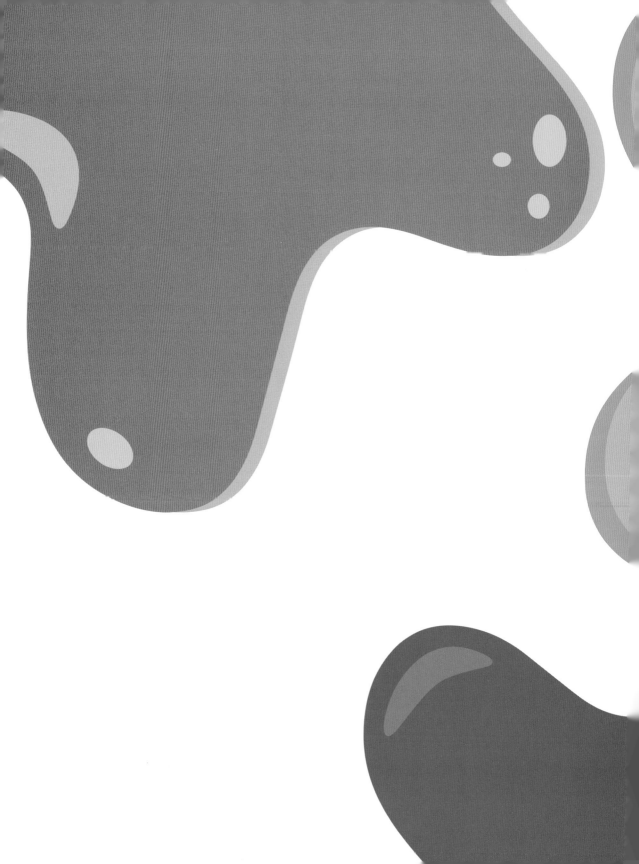

BACK SPLATTER

This section is puke-packed with bonus barf!

Since bathrooms are often the preferred place to puke, why not learn . . .

LOO LANGUAGE

Here is an international sampling of both proper and slang words for this VIP (Very Important Place).

Let's start with a classic: lavatory.

The word *lavatory* comes from the Latin word *lavo,* which means to "to wash." It once referred to a room and the washbasin in it. (A washbasin was a large bowl filled with water for washing the hands and face.) When indoor toilets became fashionable, a room with both a washbasin (a sink) and a toilet became known as a lavatory. Bathrooms on a plane are called a lavatory too.

If in your travels you find the need to "litter the loo" or "laugh at your shoes," let's make sure you know what to look for. Let's go with the flow!

badezimmer—Germany

baño—Spain

banyo—Turkey

bathroom—United States

bog—Great Britain (where you use a "bogroll," or toilet paper)

cludgie—Scotland

comfort room (or CR)—Philippines

dunny—Australia, New Zealand

gabinetto—Italian

garderobe—medieval Europe

house of office—fifteenth-century England

jacks—Ireland

john—United States

khazi—Great Britain

latrine—United States military

little girls'/boys' room—United States

loo—Great Britain

necessary room/necessary house—United States

netty—Northeast England

outhouse—United States

porta-potty—United States

powder room—United States

privy—Great Britain

restroom—United States

salle de bains—France

throne room—United States

toilet—United States

vin—England

washroom—United States

water closet (WC)—England (also France, Germany, and Mexico)

BODY PARTS

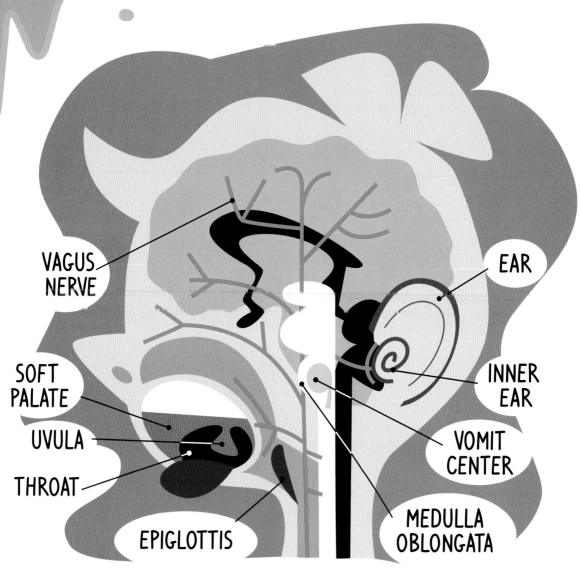

VAGUS NERVE

EAR

SOFT PALATE

UVULA

THROAT

INNER EAR

VOMIT CENTER

MEDULLA OBLONGATA

EPIGLOTTIS

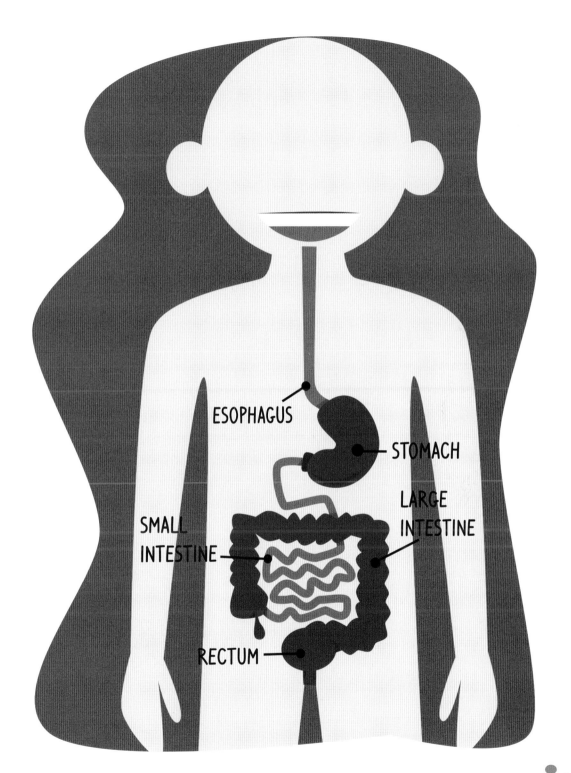

ESOPHAGUS

STOMACH

LARGE
INTESTINE

SMALL
INTESTINE

RECTUM

GLOPPY GLOSSARY

abdomen: the belly; contains the digestive organs

appendix: a small pouch attached to the top of the large intestine

bacteria: tiny organisms that can cause infection (see also *Escherichia coli*)

balance: sense of balance makes it possible for a person to know what position the body is in; an organ in the inner ear makes balance possible

bezoar: a blob of undigested food (usually) that hardens into a solid mass in the stomach, or if it gets passed through, appears somewhere else in the digestive system

bile: a greenish-yellow digestive fluid that the gallbladder stores and sends to the first part of the small intestine to help the body break down and soak up fat from food for energy

chemoreceptor trigger zone (CTZ): the area of the brain that lets the vomiting center know it's time to cause vomiting

chyme: a mushy mix of partly digested food, stomach acid, digestive enzymes, and gastric juices

contamination: when something like food becomes unsafe or unclean due to being exposed to poisons or bacteria or other harmful substances

cybersickness: happens when the brain gets conflicting information from the eyes, inner ears, joints, and muscles and doesn't know whether the person is really moving while playing video games or scrolling on a phone or other electronic device; related to motion sickness

dehydration: loss of fluid; throwing up can cause the body to lose some of the water it needs to be healthy

digestive system: the organs of the body, such as the mouth, throat, stomach, and intestines, that food and liquids travel through when they are swallowed, digested, absorbed, and leave the body

duodenum: the start of the small intestine

emesis: the process of vomiting

enteric nervous system: coordinates the process of digestion and makes it possible for the body to absorb nutrients; this system starts at the esophagus (the part that connects the throat and the stomach), then continues through the stomach and intestines and down to the anus (the very end of the large intestine where poop comes out)

epiglottis: a small "lid" made of flexible tissue called cartilage located at the base of the tongue toward the back of the throat; folds back to keep what a person eats or drinks from sliding down the windpipe when swallowing, then goes back to an upright position so that air can enter the larynx (voice box) and lungs

***Escherichia coli* (*E. coli*):** a type of bacteria that can make you sick, even if you only get a small amount in the body

from drinking contaminated water or food or from another person

esophagus: a muscular tube that lets food and drinks flow from the throat to the stomach

food poisoning: sickness caused by eating food that contains harmful bacteria or toxins, often due to improper storage or preparation

gallbladder: a part of the digestive system that stores the bile made in the liver and sends it to the stomach to help process food

gastroenteritis: an infection caused by a virus in the stomach and intestine

gastroparesis: a condition that prevents the stomach muscles from squeezing enough to move food down the digestive tract to the small intestine; signs of gastroparesis include nausea and vomiting (especially of undigested food)

glottis: the gap between your vocal cords that closes to make sure food or fluids do not go into the lungs

gluten intolerance: an inability to process gluten, which makes a person feel sick after eating the protein found in wheat and other grains (see also **lactose intolerance**)

hyperosmia: a very strong sense of smell

hypersalivation: also known as drooling; when the mouth glands make too much saliva

indigestion: an upset stomach (nausea, burping, gas) usually brought on by eating too much or too quickly

intestines (large and small): digestive organs that soak up nutrients, break down food, absorb water, and collect the waste that the body pushes out in the form of poop

kidneys: organs that remove waste from the body and make vitamin D usable for growing healthy bones

lactose intolerance: difficulty breaking down the sugars in milk, which can cause indigestion, nausea, bloating, and even vomiting after eating or drinking dairy products (see also **gluten intolerance**)

lavatory: a room with a toilet and a sink, also known as a bathroom—not to be confused with a laboratory

liver: an organ that cleans the blood leaving the stomach and intestine and sends nutrients to the rest of the body; turns leftover nutrients into a greenish-yellow digestive fluid called bile and stores it in the gallbladder

medulla oblongata: lowest part of the brain, connected to the spinal cord; manages important functions, such as keeping the lungs breathing and the heart pumping, and is home to the body's vomiting center

microbiome: a collection of trillions of microbes (bacteria, fungi, viruses, and their genes) that live on and in the body; energizes the immune system to protect the body from becoming sick, helps with digestion, and keeps harmful bacteria from growing too much

migraine: a moderate-to-severe headache that can last up to two days and come back at least a couple times a month

motion sickness: confusion between what the eyes see and what the body feels, especially the inner ear, which controls balance; can cause dizziness, nausea, and vomiting when riding in a car or on a train, airplane, boat, or amusement park ride (see also **cybersickness**)

nervous system: the body's command center; starts in the brain to control body systems, movements, and automatic responses, such as increasing the heart rate to cause the body to sweat and cool itself during vomiting

norovirus: a virus (an infectious germ that spreads by making copies of itself inside infected cells) that passes from one person to the next easily; present in the vomit (or poop) of a sick person

olfactory: the body's sensory system used for smelling

osmophobia: an extreme disgust for certain odors; can trigger a migraine headache, which can lead to nausea and vomiting

pancreas: organ located behind the stomach that makes a special enzyme (like a powerful juice) that breaks down the fat and protein in food

peristalsis: the squeezing and relaxing of muscles in the intestine that create a "wave" to keep food in the digestive system moving forward

proprioceptive system: allows your body to sense movement, tension, and pressure via joints and muscles

pyloric sphincter: a ring of smooth muscle at the lower end of the stomach that helps to move partly digested food and stomach juices into the small intestine; constricts to force vomit up and out of the gut

saliva: watery fluid that keeps the mouth moist and helps taste, chew, and swallow food, while also breaking down starches; the body makes extra saliva to protect the teeth from stomach acid when you "splurge"

uvula: a flap-like organ at the back of the throat that hangs down during breathing to send air up the nasal passage and to the lungs; when swallowing food or drink, a reflex causes the uvula to rise, closing off the nasal opening

vagus nerve: controls the muscles throughout the digestive system, so that the stomach muscles know when to push food to the digestive tract

vestibular system: inner ear, which senses movement and balance

vomiting center: the brain's "command center" for the vomiting process

CHUCK'S VOMIT VOCABULARY
in Ralphabetical Order

A

After-Dinner Drainer: when dinner goes out of you after you go out to dinner

All-Out Spout: gush grape soda like a gloppy purple geyser

Animated Throat Missiles: launch a tummy tantrum into the toilet target

Arf: barf on all fours like a dog

Atomic Vomit: when goop explodes as the belly unloads

B

Barf: arf like a dog with bad breath

Bark at the Ants: end a picnic by barfing in the basket

Belly Blowout: when the belly fills up, the belly blows out

Belly Deli: purge a pastrami and salami tsunami

Belly Jelly: un-jam food sandwiched in the stomach

Blast the Bathroom: have a belly outburst

Blow Chunks: hurl a cottage cheese smoothie

Bomb the Bathroom: explode in the commode or go kaboom in the bathroom

Boomerang Breakfast: see the return of the scrambled eggs

Burst Your Belly Bubble: eat and eat until the belly pops and lunch leaks out

C

Calling Ralph: call up an ice cream cone on the porcelain phone

Carpet the Grass: make a chuck yawn and feed the lawn

Cascade the Cat: spew kitten chow

Chew Backward: pizza goes in (chew-chew-chew), pizza comes out (ew-ew-ew)

Chew the Cheese: hurl an absurd pile of curds

Chuck: toss the anchovy pizza sauce

Chuckle on the Bus: the meals in the gut go round and round

Chum Bucket: *see* fish salad swish

Chunder: the rumble of thunder down under before the brekky (Aussie for breakfast) rains into the dunny (toilet)

Chunk: dunk a pukey hunk that stinks like a skunk

Clean House: plop stomach slop, stop, and then mop

Collywobbles: nervous tummy rumbles followed by a chunder storm

D

Decorate the Doorknob: splatter the door, then three times more

Deliver Groceries: bag eggs, bread, and milk in the belly—then drop them at the bathroom door

Dinner to Go: when you dine and the dinner dashes

Download Dinner: transfer the bile file to "commode overflowed" code

Drive the Porcelain Bus: grab the toilet-seat-shaped steering wheel while the bus is unloading

Drown Your Desk: sit in science class and see a notebook swimming in gut goop

Dry Heave: honk hot air as you stare at the toilet down there

Dunk: drop damp doughnuts, as in "Hey, Queezy, downing a dozen jelly doughnuts after soccer will make me dunk!"

E

Earp: swiftly slurp, then burp and blow

Eat Backward: chew through a ton of cashews and then they come back to you

Elevator: send lunch for a ride from the belly floor to the top floor

Emergency Stomach Evacuation: when the stomach calls "Everybody exit!"

Emesis Me: dribble barf down the belly

Erupting Grocery Geyser: eat every treat your parent brought home from the store before the gut tosses them back in the bag

Exit Emesis: direct the snack to the nearest exit

Face Fountain: feel pink lemonade and orange soda flow down your frown

Fast Food: when you see (and feel) your sausage sandwich speed away

Feed the Fishes: let the minnows munch your pre-munched lunch

Flash: when your dinner decides to dash

Flounder: when your stomach flips and your fish dinner flops

Food Fire Drill: eat spicy rice and feel it head for the emergency exit

Forge Ahead: where mashed potatoes meet water gravy

Free Soup: when your misery makes a big bowl of mystery

Frothy Cough: foam root beer float from your face

Gag: when you dry heave to relieve the zig-zag-do-I-need-a-barf-bag nag in the gut

Gargle Gravy: pack away mashed potatoes, then spew your spuds

Goodbye Pie: feel flaky before the crusty dessert deserts you

Goop: ploop out soggy soup

Gunk: what you hurl from the trunk

Gurp: belch up a spinach smoothie

Gush: hurl slush and rush to flush

Gut Grief: when you wolf down a sidewalk pizza (or six) and a whole Barfday Cake

Gut Soup: spew stomach slop with crumbled crackers

H

Hack: unpack the gooey gut sack

Hawk Your Head Off: hurl food with such force, your face goes flying

Heading Out: when squishy food spurts up your throat and out your mouth hole

Heave Up Jonah: open wide like a whale with a salty Jonah ready to bail

Hoist Your Toenails: heave so hard you end up with toes for teeth

Hold the Throne: hold the phone while you fill the throne

Holler: open wide and yell out the yuck

Honk Hot Air: when spicy food calls a fire drill and shoots flames out the face

Hoop: feel what was turning around in the belly roll on out

Hork: when you got a bit too piggy with the pork and spew barbecue

Hughie: spewy in the loo-y

Hurl: feel the food whirl and unfurl out of your face

I

Ill Will: feel nauseous waiting to see what the stomach will do

Insides Out: when you go out to lunch, and then lunch goes out on you

Insult the Shoes: leak lasagna and splurt spaghetti on your sandals

Interesting Outcome: see what a taco looks like turned inside out

Interior Desecrator: move your stomach's interior to your shirt's exterior

Interrupting Eruption: when your belly bubbles over and breakfast bursts out

Irresistible Purge: when you can't stop unstuffing your stomach

J

Jelly Belly: jam the belly with too much jelly ("Oops. I made something smelly.")

Jiggly Juice: produce a jiggly pool of cottage cheese and tomato juice

Juggle Jambalaya: stuff yourself with a spicy, ricey mishmash until the belly balks and you spew into the bayou

Jumble Juice: when orange juice pours out your face spout

Jump Shot: when puke bypasses the toilet and detours to the tub

K

Kaleidoscope Cough: spew a colorful swirl of oranges, blueberries, and green beans

Keep It Moving: bring breakfast back

Kneel Before the Porcelain Throne: bow in front of the barfing bowl

Knock-Knock! Spew's There?: Spew who? Spew better move!

L

Laugh at Your Shoes: liquefy the laces and soak your funny-looking socks

Leftovers and Out: when the eggs scramble in the stomach and wrestle to be free-range

Liquid Scream: stream ice cream like a bad dream

Litter the Loo: when you set free a deep-dish debris spree ("I thought pizza was my friend.")

Lose Your Lunch: bag up the midday meal and unpack it all over the lunch table

Lumpy Burp: when meatballs retreat and return as *repeat*-balls

Lurch: when your lunch goes out to launch

M

Make a Chunky Puddle: cough up mac and cheese and chocolate milk on the crosswalk

Meal-to-Go: when breakfast goes from a takeout bag to a barf bag

Meh Overboard: vomit, but, eh, so what? As in "So I made a chunky puddle. Meh. No big deal."

Messy Middle: when what's inside the middle of you spews down the front of you

Moist Hoist: feel the stomach foist funky tofu

Move Out: pack away pie and have it escape for another try

Mustard Mash: hurl yellowish-green goo after a hot dog or two (or six)

My Lunch Says Hello: bid your burrito goodbye, but then it rebounds

No-Brainer Gut Drainer: before you have a chance to blink, your burrito's in the sink

Nonstop Glop: when the vomit hits repeat

Noot: poke fruit down the shoot and feel a dispute before the gut gives that fruit the boot ("Wah! I liked that kiwi!")

Nose Way: puke out the proboscis (also known as the nose!)

Nowhere to Hide: when the gut puts your gut groceries all out there

Nurffle: overfill, then feel ill till you spill

Oodles o' Noodles: what happens when spaghetti is ready to retreat, as in "Oops. My pasta popped out. I made oodles o' noodles!"

Open Wide for What's Inside: when the fried squid you tried slides back outside

Out Spout: churn out vomit from the snout

Over and Out: gross out when leftover brussels sprouts abruptly leak out

Overweight Burp: belch with a hefty surprise ending

Paint the Walls: when stomach matter climbs up the ladder to splatter and scatter

Park at the Porcelain Pool: when puke uses the tongue for a diving board

Pavement Pizza: deliver pepperoni and extra cheese to the sidewalk

Perk: when the belly becomes alert because it's about to spurt

Plornk: plunk the potbelly's bloat overboard

Plummet: catapult a plum (or six) from the tum

Pour the Punch: purge purple party punch in the bowl

Puddle Pudding: when curdled custard spurts like mustard

Puke: revisit your rigatoni, ramen, rice, or macaroni

Quack: when your snack ducks out

Quaggy Gaggy: time for the mushy to go flushy

Quake and Shake: shiver and quiver while barfing onions and liver

Quark: quack in the park after dark (see also **Quack**)

Queasy Sneezy: when your stomach feels full of meatball yo-yos and you "sneeze" all over the pillows

Quick Getaway: when dessert decides to dash

Quick Sick: when you had a quack-free shirt a split second before (see also **Quack**)

Rainbow Retch: top off the porcelain pot at the end of the rainbow

Ralph: Ruth

Ralph on a Roller Coaster: fill up, then feel down when the stomach does a corkscrew

Recall: bring a meal back after the buffet

Restroom Karaoke: sing into the potty after too much pizza at a party

Return for a Refund: purchase a meal, eat it, and have it come back on you

Reverse Gears: when wheels in the gut go round and round the wrong way

Rup: have a belly ready to burst, as in "Stand back! He's ready to rup!"

Ruth: Ralph (see also **Ralph on a Roller Coaster**)

Seasick: go for a boat ride and hurl over the side

Secondhand Dinner: see supper inside out

Set Lunch Free: open the gate and let the burger bolt ("Hey! Now that's fast food!")

Shoot Soup: slurp it all in and spout it all out

Sick: feel unwell, out of sorts, woozy, and green after eating an unclean tangerine

Sling Everything: fling a belly full

Slorge: what happens after you gorge and go all Curious George on bananas

Spewing Spree: feel sushi go splooshy

Spewnami: ride a rolling wave of vomit with an undercurrent of nausea

Spill the Soup: fill the potbelly with chowder, then move it out-er

Spit Up: receive a free sample of the slop to come

Surf the Wave: when you feel stoked, but the stomach feels provoked ("Dude! Hang loose! My gut wants to wipe out!")

T

Technicolor Yawn: open wide and let the rainbow flow to the bathroom bowl

Throw Up: after a cup of cheese soup, the gut winds up, then blows up . . . heads up!

Tip the Shopping Cart: when groceries roll up on the belly's conveyor belt

Toilet Yodel: overeat Swiss cheese and blow it out your yodel hole

Tonsil Toss: feel the loss of the applesauce as it shoots across the tonsils

Toss Your Tacos: when you hear lunch say "vamos" (let's go) and then it does ("Bye! Sad to see you go, tacos!")

Tummy Tantrum: when the belly blows up and tosses tofu in the toilet

U

Uncap the Queso: send the spicy nachos on a trip

Un-Food: feel food in your stomach dash for the nearest exit

Unleash the Monster: spew an ogre out of your innards

Unpack: come home from camp and drop a load of dirty socks

Up and Out: when the food that's been down-and-in celebrates Opposite Day ("I wish my dinner did the opposite!")

Upchuck: muck out the yuck that's stuck in the middle

Urp: the surprise of a burp with a bonus

Vaulting Vittles: when what's in your middle leaps over the tongue

Vent Gross Grub: release greasy gobs from your belly blobs

Vile Veggie Vacation: produce a glistening pool of broccoli, beets, and tomato juice

Visit Barfville: drop by the world's grossest rest stop and leave a souvenir

Vombination Unlock: when your body uses the right combination to empty the vault

Vombo Combo: when peanut butter and jelly from the deli mix with pickles in the belly ("Who ordered takeout?")

Vomcano: expel lunch-ish-looking lava from your mouth

Vomit: drop the waffles off at the whirlpool ("Whee!")

Voomerang: when you finish a snack only to have it come back around

Waah: hurl so hard you make your stomach sob

Waves of Woe: vomit not once but repeatedly, while sailing stormy seas ("Abandon ship!")

Wear Your Lunch: what happens when vomit makes you a whole new outfit

Wet Burp: learn what an inside-out wet burrito looks like ("Dude. I cannot unsee that.")

Whistle Chunks: blow barf for all to hear

Whoa: Hold on to the sink! What's that pink stink? ("Did you eat the whole watermelon?")

Whoopsie: when you aim for the bowl but miss the whole hole

Woop: slip out a sloppy scoop of goopy gut soup, as in "Oops. I wooped my boots."

Xanthic Banana Barf: produce pale, yellowish spit-up scented with banana

X-It Up: send chewed food, which was once down, up and out again

X Marks the Spot: find the perfect place to puke

X-plosive Exports: push peppery puke out the mouth port

X-treme Emesis: vomit so hard, so loud, and so long that you'll tell the grandchildren about it one day

Yack Your Snack: return a liquefied lunch into your backpack

Yarf: explode the whole of it, not the harf (half) of it

Yawp: cry for yelp (help) after slurping down kelp

Yeech: hawk up a peach—pit and all—on the beach

Yell at the Ground: shout slop at the floor

Yodel Your Lunch: set the cheesy fondue free in Switzerland ("Ew. My song came out wrong!")

Yo-Yo: what goes down . . . may come up . . . then down (and all over!)

Yuck: disgust even yourself

Yurk: go berserk and hurl a ham on rye at the homework ("Sorry, Ms. Snard. I yurked my homework.")

Z

Zilch: spew until there's zero left in your stomach

Zink: empty the contents of your stomach in the kitchen ("I had to zink in the sink.")

Zombie Zarf: barf your brains out

Zool: hurl into a body of water ("I had to zool in the pool.")

Zoo Spew: when the vomit smells like petting zoo poo

Zork: drop your fork and let your fish sticks fly

Zowerswop: sip so much zippy zuppa, it comes back uppa

Zuke: puke for the last time (that day), as in "My belly is zuked out."

Zutter: accidentally inhale a butterfly and barf it up

ACKNOWLEDGMENTS

My overflowing gratitude:

To my ever-encouraging parents, Wayne and Cassie Mueller; to my late grandmother Frances Wilkinson, who showed me how to have fun with words; and to my priceless children, Ryan and Ann-Marie. You inspire me to persevere. I can only hope to make you half as proud as you make me.

To my exceptional editor, Tom Russell. You made this entire experience a joy. Thank you for inviting my input throughout the spew-tiful creative process, and to the beyond-amazing "behind the scenes" team at Bright Matter Books: Eugenia Lo, Publishing Assistant; Rebecca Vitkus, Managing Editor; Alison Kolani, Copy Editor; and Michelle Crowe, Designer.

To the unforgettable "Barfmeister" Brett Wright, who shares my love of painful puns. Thank you, thank you, thank you for seeing what this book could be and for all you did to get it there.

To my brilliant illustrator, Remy Simard, who captured my silly characters so perfectly. I admire your capacity for collaboration and your delightful artistic skills.

To my agent extraordinaire, Erin Murphy, for being my champion and cheerleader (and sometimes counselor). I am beyond thankful for you. xo

To my faithful friends Kris Remenar, Ruth McNally Barshaw, and Charlie Barshaw, for your invaluable notes when *The Big Book of Barf* was but a bitty booklet, and for your boundless enthusiasm to this day; and to my many (many!) steadfast encouragers, including Kelly Barson, Ann Finkelstein, Hope Vestergaard, and Susan Wilkinson, for your uncanny ability to make me laugh through tears and help me find the courage to try again, and again. . . .

To the Michigan chapter of the Society of Children's Book Writers and Illustrators (SCBWI). Thanks to a 2020 SCBWI-MI workshop, I learned how to create a nonfiction book proposal. (Guess what? It worked!)

And finally, to two of the bravest kids I know—my fearless recipe testers: Ben and Sofia Hall. I owe you a triple-decker Barfday Cake!

Because I am fearfully and wonderfully made.
I know that full well.
Psalm 139:14

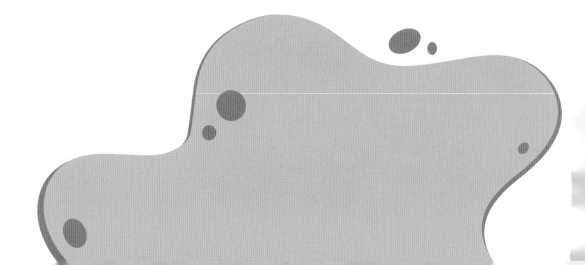

ABOUT THE AUTHOR

Becoming a children's author has been Vicky Lorencen's lifelong dream. En route to achieving that, Vicky's been a college writing instructor and a freelance journalist, and for the last fifteen years, she's been in healthcare communications, writing about everything from allergies to Zika virus. Her work for young readers has appeared in *Highlights for Children, Ladybug,* and *Girls' Life.* Vicky and her husband live in Michigan, where she runs a summer day camp for dust bunnies. Visit her at VickyLorencen.com.